MW00679571

DSM-IV DRAFT CRITERIA

3/1/93

TASK FORCE ON DSM-IV

American Psychiatric Association

Copyright 1993 by the American Psychiatric Association, 1400 K Street, N.W.,
Washington, D.C. 20005

Table of Contents

DSM-IV Task Force and Staff
Acknowledgments
Preface

A: Introduction to DSM-IV and Cautionary Statement
B: Use of the Manual
C: DSM-IV Classification
D: Multiaxial Assessment
E: Disorders Usually First Diagnosed in Infancy, Childhood, or Adolescence
F: Delirium, Dementia, Amnestic and Other Cognitive Disorders
G: Mental Disorders Due to a General Medical Condition
H: Substance-Related Disorders
I: Schizophrenia and Other Psychotic Disorders
J: Mood Disorders
K: Anxiety Disorders
L: Somatoform Disorders
M: Factitious Disorders
N: Dissociative Disorders
O: Sexual and Gender Identity Disorders
P: Eating Disorders
Q: Sleep Disorders
R: Impulse Control Disorders Not Elsewhere Classified
S: Adjustment Disorder
T: Personality Disorders
U: Other Conditions That May Be a Focus of Clinical Attention
V: Additional Codes
W: DSM-IV Appendices
X: Afterword

Task Force on DSM-IV

Allen Frances, M.D., Chair
Nancy Andreasen, M.D., Ph.D.
David Barlow, Ph.D.
Magda Campbell, M.D.
Dennis Cantwell, M.D.
Ellen Frank, Ph.D.
Judith Gold, M.D.
John Gunderson M.D.
Robert Hales, M.D.
Kenneth Kendler, M.D.
David Kupfer, M.D.
Michael Liebowitz, M.D.
Juan Mezzich, M.D.
Peter Nathan, Ph.D.
Roger Peele, M.D.
Darrel A. Regier, M.D.
A. John Rush, M.D.
Chester Schmidt, M.D.
Marc Schuckit, M.D.
David Shaffer, M.D.
Robert L. Spitzer, M.D., Special Advisor
Gary Tucker, M.D.
John Urbaitis, M.D., Assembly Liaison
B. Timothy Walsh, M.D.
Janet B.W. Williams, D.S.W.

James Hudziak, M.D., APA Resident Fellow (1990-92)
Junius Gonzalez, M.D., APA Resident Fellow (1988-90)

DSM-IV Staff

Harold Alan Pincus, M.D., APA Deputy Medical Director
Michael B. First, M.D., Editor, Text and Criteria
Thomas Widiger, Ph.D., Research Coordinator
Ruth Ross, M.A., Science Writer
Wendy Davis, Ed.M., Editorial Coordinator
Nancy Vettorello, M.U.P., Administrative Coordinator
Nancy Sydnor-Greenberg, M.A., Administrative Coordinator
Myriam Kline, M.S., Focused Field Trial Coordinator
James Thompson, M.D., Videotape Field Trial Coordinator
Cindy Jones, DSM-IV Assistant

Acknowledgments

DSM-IV is a team effort. More than 1000 people (and numerous professional organizations) have helped us in the preparation of this document. Unfortunately, space constraints prevent us from giving adequate recognition for all of these efforts. A comprehensive list of participants, noting their specific contributions, will be included both in DSM-IV and in the DSM-IV Sourcebook.

The major responsibility for the content of DSM-IV rests with the Task Force on DSM-IV and Members of the DSM-IV Work Groups. They have worked (often much harder than they bargained for) with a dedication and good cheer that has been inspirational to us. Bob Spitzer has our special thanks for his untiring efforts and unique perspective. Norman Sartorius, Darrel Regier, Lewis Judd, Fred Goodwin, and Chuck Kaelber were instrumental in facilitating a mutually productive interchange between the APA and the World Health Organization that has improved both DSM-IV and ICD-10, and increased their compatibility. We are grateful to Robert Israel at the National Center for Health Statistics and Andrea Albaum-Feinstein at the American Health Information Management Association for suggestions on the DSM-IV coding system. Denis Prager, Peter Nathan, and David Kupfer helped us in developing a novel data reanalysis strategy that has been supported with funding from the John C. and Catherine T. MacArthur Foundation.

There are several individuals within the APA who deserve recognition. Mel Sabshin's special wisdom and grace made even the most tedious tasks seem worth doing. The APA Committee on Diagnosis and Assessment (chaired by Layton McCurdy) provided valuable direction and counsel. We would also like to thank the APA Presidents (Drs. Fink, Pardes, Benedek, Hartmann, English, and McIntyre) and Assembly Speakers (Drs. Cohen, Flamm, Hanin, Pfaehler, and Shellow) who helped with the planning of our work. Carolyn Robinowitz and Jack White, and their respective staffs in the APA Medical Director's Office and the Business Office, have provided valuable assistance in the organization of the project.

Several other individuals have our special gratitude. Wendy Davis, Nancy Vettorello, and Nancy Sydnor-Greenberg developed and implemented an organizational structure that has kept this complex project from spinning out of control. We have also been blessed with an unusually able administrative staff, which has included Willa Hall, Kelly McKinney, Gloria Miele, Helen Stayna, Sarah Tilly, Nina Rosenthal, Susan Mann, Joanne Mas, and especially Cindy Jones. Ruth Ross has been responsible for improving the clarity of expression and organization of DSM-IV. Myriam Kline (Research Coordinator for the NIH-funded DSM-IV Focused Field Trials), Jim Thompson (Research Coordinator for the MacArthur Foundation-funded Videotape Field Trial), and Sandy Ferris (Administrative Coordinator for the Office of Research) have made many valuable contributions. Ron McMillen, Claire Reinburg, and Pam Harley have provided expert production assistance.

Allen Frances, M.D.
Chair, DSM-IV Task Force

Harold Alan Pincus, M.D.
APA Deputy Medical Director

Michael B. First, M.D.
Editor, DSM-IV Text and Criteria

Thomas A. Widiger, Ph.D.
Research Coordinator

Preface

This volume contains a draft of the DSM-IV criteria sets as of 3/1/93. Its contents are the culmination of more than four years of effort that have included: 1) a systematic review of the existing literature; 2) reanalyses of available data sets; 3) focused field trials that evaluated the performance of a number of the criteria sets; 4) consideration of critiques on the Options Book (published 9/1/91) and of subsequent drafts of criteria sets; 5) publication of many journal articles and a DSM-IV newsletter to keep the broadest array of individuals informed about our progress; 6) presentations of the work in progress at professional meetings; 7) extensive interaction with the American Psychiatric Association's (APA) Committee on Diagnosis and Assessment, the APA Council on Research, and other APA governance committees and components; 8) consultation with other health and mental health organizations; and 9) input from more than one thousand clinicians and researchers in the United States and abroad. Our major goals in revising the criteria have been to enhance the clinical utility of DSM-IV, to increase its empirical foundation, to maintain full compatibility with the International Classification of Diseases, and to be conservative in making changes. This draft of the criteria sets is offered as a likely near-final version, pending final consideration and approval by the APA Assembly of District Branches and Board of Trustees.

Also included in this volume are draft versions of the DSM-IV chapters "Introduction to DSM-IV," "Use of the Manual," and "Multiaxial Assessment." We are currently working towards completing the texts for each of the DSM-IV disorders and are compiling the DSM-IV Appendices. If all goes as planned, DSM-IV should be published in late 1993 or early 1994.

Introduction to DSM-IV

This is the fourth edition of the American Psychiatric Association's Diagnostic and Statistical Manual of Mental Disorders, or DSM-IV. The utility and credibility of DSM-IV require that it focus upon its clinical, research and educational purposes and be supported by an extensive empirical foundation. Our highest priority has been to provide a useful guide to clinical practice. We hoped to make DSM-IV practical and useful for clinicians by striving for brevity of criteria sets, clarity of language, and explicit statements of the constructs embodied in the diagnostic criteria. An additional goal was to facilitate research and improve communication between clinicians and researchers. We were also mindful of the use of DSM-IV for improving the collection of clinical information and as an educational tool for teaching psychopathology.

An official nomenclature must be applicable to the widest diversity of contexts in which it is used. DSM-IV is used by clinicians and researchers of many different orientations (e.g., biological, psychodynamic, cognitive, behavioral, interpersonal, family/systems). It is used by psychiatrists, other physicians, psychologists, social workers, nurses, occupational and rehabilitation therapists, counselors, and other health and mental health professionals. DSM-IV must be usable across settings--inpatients, outpatient, partial hospital, consultation/liaison, clinic, private practice, and primary care, and with community populations. It is also a necessary tool for collecting and communicating accurate public health statistics. Fortunately, all these many uses are usually compatible with one another.

DSM-IV was the product of 13 Work Groups (see page xx), each of which had primary responsibility for a section in the manual. This organization was designed to increase participation by experts in each of the respective fields. We took a number of precautions to ensure that the Work Group recommendations would reflect the breadth of available evidence and opinion and not just the views of the specific members. After extensive consultations with experts and clinicians in each field, we selected Work Group members who represented a wide range of perspectives and experiences. Work Group members were instructed that they were to participate as consensus scholars and not as advocates of previously held views. Furthermore, we established a formal evidence-based process for the Work Groups to follow.

The Work Groups reported to the DSM-IV Task Force (see page xx), consisting of of 27 members, many of whom also chaired a Work Group. Each of the 13 Work Groups was composed of five to eight members whose reviews were critiqued by between 50 and 100 advisers who were also chosen to represent diverse clinical and research expertise, disciplines, backgrounds, and settings. The involvement of many international experts ensured that DSM-IV had available the widest pool of data and would be applicable across cultures. Conferences and workshops were held to provide conceptual and methodological guidance and support for the DSM-IV effort. These included many conferences and consultations to promote ICD/DSM compatibility; and conferences that were focused on cultural factors in psychiatric diagnosis, on geriatric diagnosis, and on psychiatric diagnosis in primary care settings.

In order to maintain open and extensive lines of communication, the DSM-IV Task Force established a liaison with many other components within the American Psychiatric Association and with more than sixty organizations and associations interested in the development of DSM-IV (e.g., the World Health Organization, the National Center for Health Statistics, the American Health Information Management Association, the American Psychoanalytic Association, the American Psychological Association, the American Psychological Society, the National Association of Social Workers, the American Nursing Association, the American Occupational Therapy Association, the Coalition for the Family, the Group for the Advancement of Psychiatry). We attempted to air issues and empirical evidence early in the process in order to identify potential problems and differences in interpretation. Exchanges of information were also made possible through the distribution of a semi-annual newsletter (the DSM-IV Update), the publication of a regular column on DSM-IV in Hospital and Community Psychiatry, frequent presentations at national and international conferences, and numerous journal articles.

Two years before the publication of DSM-IV, the Task Force published and widely distributed the DSM-IV Options Book. This volume presented a comprehensive summary of the alternative proposals that were being considered for inclusion in DSM-IV in order to solicit opinion and additional data for our deliberations. We received extensive correspondence from interested individuals who shared with us additional data and recommendations on the potential impact of the possible changes in DSM-IV on their clinical practice, teaching, research, and administrative work. This breadth of discussion helped us to anticipate problems and attempt to find the best solution among the various options. One year before the publication of DSM-IV, a near-final draft of the proposed criteria sets was distributed in order to allow for one last critique.

In arriving at final DSM-IV decisions, the Work Groups and Task Force reviewed all of the extensive empirical evidence and correspondence that had been gathered. It is our belief that the major innovation of DSM-IV lies not in any of its specific content changes but rather in the systematic and explicit process by which it was constructed and documented. More than any other nomenclature of mental disorders, DSM-IV is grounded in empirical evidence.

HISTORICAL BACKGROUND

The need for a classification of mental disorders has been clear throughout the history of medicine, but there has been little agreement on the optimal method for organizing disorders and which disorders should be included. The many nomenclatures that have been developed during the past two millennia have differed in their relative emphasis on phenomenology, etiology, and course as defining features. Some systems have included only a handful of diagnostic categories; others have included thousands. Moreover, the various systems for categorizing mental disorders have differed with respect to whether their principle objective was for use in clinical, research, or statistical settings. Because the history of classification is too extensive to be summarized here, we will focus briefly only on those aspects that have led directly to the development of the Diagnostic and Statistical Manual of Mental Disorders (DSM) and to the Mental Disorders section of the International Classification of Diseases (ICD).

In the United States, the initial impetus for developing a classification of mental disorders was the need to collect statistical information. What might be considered the first official attempt to gather information about mental illness in the U.S. was the recording of the frequency of one category--"idiocy/insanity" in the 1840 census. By the 1880 census, seven categories were distinguished (mania, melancholia, monomania, paresis, dementia, dipsomania, and epilepsy). In 1917 the Committee on Statistics of the American Psychiatric Association formulated a plan that was adopted by the Bureau of the Census for gathering uniform statistics across mental hospitals. Although this system devoted more attention to clinical utility than did previous systems, it was still primarily a statistical classification. The APA subsequently collaborated with the New York Academy of Medicine to develop a nationally acceptable psychiatric nomenclature that would be incorporated within the first edition of the American Medical Association's Standard Classified Nomenclature of Disease. This nomenclature was designed primarily for diagnosing inpatients suffering from severe psychiatric and neurological disorders.

A much broader nomenclature was later developed by the U.S. Army (and modified by the Veterans Administration) in order to better incorporate the outpatient presentations of World War II servicemen and veterans (e.g., psychophysiological, personality, and acute disorders). Contemporaneously, the World Health Organization (WHO) published the sixth edition of the International Classification of Diseases (ICD) which, for the first time, included a section for mental disorders. ICD-6 was heavily influenced by the Veterans Administration nomenclature and included ten categories for psychoses, nine for psychoneuroses, and seven for disorders of character, behavior, and intelligence.

The APA Committee on Nomenclature and Statistics developed a variant of the ICD-6 that was published in 1952 as the first edition of the Diagnostic and Statistical Manual, Mental Disorders (DSM-I). DSM-I contained a glossary of descriptions of the diagnostic categories and was the first official manual of mental disorders to focus on clinical utility. The use of the term reaction throughout DSM-I reflected the influence of Adolf Meyer's psychobiologic view that mental disorders represented reactions of the personality to psychological, social, and biological factors.

In part because of the lack of widespread acceptance of the mental disorder taxonomy contained in ICD-6 and ICD-7, the WHO sponsored a comprehensive review of diagnostic issues which was conducted by the British psychiatrist Stengel. His report can be credited with having inspired many of the recent advances in diagnostic methodology--most especially the need for explicit definitions as a means of promoting reliable clinical diagnoses. However, the next round of diagnostic revision, which led to DSM-II and ICD-8, did not follow Stengel's recommendations to any great degree. DSM-II was similar to DSM-I but eliminated the use of the term "reaction."

As had been the case for DSM-I and DSM-II, the development of DSM-III was coordinated with the development of the next (ninth) version of the ICD, which was published in 1975 and implemented in 1978. Work began on DSM-III in 1974, with publication in 1980. DSM-III introduced a number of important methodological innovations, including explicit diagnostic criteria, a multiaxial system, and a descriptive approach that attempted to be neutral with respect to theories of etiology. This effort was facilitated by the extensive empirical work then underway on the construction and validation of explicit diagnostic criteria and the development of semistructured interviews. The ICD-9 did not include diagnostic criteria or a multiaxial system largely because the primary function of this international system was the classification of morbidity in the collection of basic health statistics. In contrast, DSM-III was developed with the additional goal of providing a medical nomenclature for clinicians and researchers. Because of dissatisfaction across all of medicine with the lack of specificity in ICD-9, a decision was made to modify it for use in the United States by expanding the four-digit ICD-9 codes to the five-digit ICD-9-CM (for Clinical Modification) codes which permitted greater specificity. This made it possible for the DSM-III classification and virtually all of its diagnostic terms to be included in the ICD-9-CM classification.

Experience with DSM-III had revealed a number of inconsistencies in the system and a number of instances in which the criteria were not entirely clear. Therefore, the APA appointed a Work Group to Revise DSM-III which made the revisions and corrections that led to the publication of DSM-III-R in 1987.

THE DSM-IV REVISION PROCESS

The third edition of the Diagnostic and Statistical Manual of Mental Disorders (DSM-III) represented a major advance in the diagnosis of mental disorder and greatly facilitated empirical research. The development of DSM-IV has benefitted from the substantial increase in the research on diagnosis that was generated in part by DSM-III and DSM-III-R. Most diagnoses now have an empirical literature or available data sets that are relevant to decisions regarding the revision of the diagnostic manual. The Task Force on DSM-IV and its Work Groups have conducted a three-stage empirical process that includes: 1) comprehensive and systematic reviews of the published literature, 2) reanalyses of already-collected data sets, and 3) extensive issue-focused field trials.

Literature Reviews: We sponsored two methods conferences to articulate for all the Work Groups a systematic procedure for finding, extracting, aggregating, and interpreting data in a comprehensive and objective fashion. The initial task of each of the DSM-IV Work Groups was to identify the most pertinent issues regarding each diagnosis and to determine the kinds of empirical data relevant to their resolution. A Work Group member or adviser was then assigned the responsibility of conducting a systematic and comprehensive review of the relevant literature that would inform the resolution of the issue and also document the text of DSM-IV. The domains considered in making decisions included clinical utility, reliability, descriptive validity, the performance characteristics of individual criteria, and a number of validating variables.

Each literature review specified: (1) the issues or aspects of the text under consideration and the significance of the issues with respect to the DSM; (2) the review method (including the sources for identifying relevant studies, the criteria for inclusion and exclusion from the review, the number of studies considered, and the variables catalogued in each study); (3) the results of the review (including a descriptive summary of the studies with respect to methodology, design, and substantive correlates of the findings; the relevant findings; and the analyses conducted on these findings); and (4) the various options for resolving the issue, the advantages and disadvantages of each option, recommendations, and any additional research that would be needed to provide a more conclusive resolution.

The goal of the DSM-IV literature reviews was to be comprehensive and unbiased. For this reason, we used systematic computer searches and critiques done by a large group of advisers to ensure that the literature coverage was adequate and the interpretation of the results justified. Input was solicited especially from those persons likely to be critical of the conclusions of the review. The literature reviews were revised many times to ensure that they were sufficiently comprehensive and balanced. It must be noted that for some issues addressed by the DSM-IV Work Groups, particularly those that were more conceptual in nature or for which there were insufficient data, a review of the empirical literature had limited utility. Despite these limitations, the reviews were helpful in ensuring that DSM-IV reflects the best available clinical and research literature and in documenting the rationale and empirical support for decisions made by the DSM-IV Work Groups.

Data reanalysis: When a review of the literature revealed a lack of evidence (or conflicting evidence) for the resolution of an issue, we often made use of two additional resources, data reanalyses and field trials, to help in making final decisions. Analyses of existing and relevant unpublished data sets were supported by a grant to the American Psychiatric Association from the John D. and Catherine T. MacArthur Foundation. Most of the 40 data reanalyses performed for DSM-IV involved the collaboration of several investigators at different sites. These researchers jointly subjected their data to questions posed by the Work Groups concerning the criteria included in DSM-III-R or criteria that might be included in DSM-IV. Data reanalyses also made it possible for Work Groups to generate several data-based criteria sets. These sets were then tested in the DSM-IV field trials. Although, for the most part, the data sets used in the reanalyses had been collected as part of epidemiological, treatment, or other clinical studies, they were also highly relevant to the nosological questions facing the DSM-IV Work Groups.

Field Trials: The 12 DSM-IV field trials were sponsored by the National Institute of Mental Health (NIMH) in collaboration with the National Institute on Drug Abuse (NIDA) and the National Institute on Alcohol Abuse and Alcoholism (NIAAA). The field trials allowed the DSM-IV Work Groups to compare alternative options and to study the possible impact of suggested changes. Field trials compared DSM-III, DSM-III-R, ICD-10, and proposed DSM-IV criteria sets in 5 to 10 different sites with approximately 100 subjects at each site. Diverse sites, with representative groups of subjects from a range of sociocultural and ethnic backgrounds, were selected to ensure generalizability of field trial results and to test some of the most difficult questions in differential diagnosis. The 12 field trials included more than 70 sites and evaluated more than 6000 subjects. The field trials collected information on the reliability and performance characteristics of each criteria set as a whole as well as of the specific items within each criteria set. Field trials also helped to bridge the boundary between clinical research and clinical practice by determining how well suggestions for change derived from clinical research findings apply in clinical practice.

Criteria for Change: Although it was impossible to develop absolute and infallible criteria for when changes should be made, there were some principles that guided our efforts. The threshold for making revisions in DSM-IV was set higher than for DSM-III and DSM-III-R. Decisions had to be substantiated by explicit statements of rationale and by the systematic review of relevant empirical data. In order to increase the practicality and clinical utility of DSM-IV, the criteria sets were simplified and clarified when this could be justified by empirical data. There was an attempt to strike an optimal balance in DSM-IV with respect to historical tradition (as embodied in DSM-III and DSM-III-R), compatibility with ICD-10, evidence from reviews of the literature, unpublished data sets, field trials, and consensus of the field. Although the requirement for evidence to support changes was set high, it necessarily varied across disorders because the empirical support for the decisions made in DSM-III and DSM-III-R also varied across disorders. Of course, common sense was necessary and major changes solving minor problems required more evidence than minor changes solving major problems.

We received suggestions that numerous possible new diagnoses be included in DSM-IV. The proponents argued that the new diagnoses were necessary to improve the coverage of the system by including a group of individuals currently undiagnosable in DSM-III-R or diagnosable only under the Not Otherwise Specified rubric. We decided that, in general, new diagnoses should be included in the system only after they have proven themselves through research rather than being included to stimulate that research. However, diagnoses already included in ICD-10 were given somewhat more consideration than those that were being introduced fresh for DSM-IV. The increased marginal utility, clarity, and coverage provided by each newly proposed diagnosis had to be balanced against the cumulative cumbersomeness imposed on the whole system, the lack of empirical documentation, and the possible misdiagnosis or misuse that might result. No classification of mental disorders can have a sufficient number of specific categories to encompass every conceivable presentation. Therefore the NOS categories are provided to cover the not infrequent presentation that is at the boundary of specific categorical definitions.

The DSM-IV Sourcebook: Documentation has been the essential foundation of the DSM-IV process. The DSM-IV Sourcebook, published in five volumes, is intended to provide a comprehensive and convenient reference record of the clinical and research support for the various decisions reached by the Work Groups and Task Force. The first three volumes of the DSM-IV Sourcebook contain condensed versions of the 150 DSM-IV literature reviews. The fourth volume contains reports of the data reanalyses, and the fifth volume contains reports of the field trials and a final executive summary of the rationale for the decisions made by each Work Group. In addition, many papers were stimulated by the efforts towards empirical documentation in DSM-IV and these have been published in peer-reviewed journals.

Relation to ICD-10: The tenth revision of the International Classification of Diseases (ICD-10), developed by the World Health Organization, was published in 1992, but will probably not become official in the United States until the late 1990s. Those preparing the ICD-10 and DSM-IV have worked closely to coordinate their efforts, resulting in much mutual influence. The ICD-10 consists of an official coding system and other related clinical and research documents and instruments. The codes and terms provided in DSM-IV are fully compatible with both ICD-9-CM and ICD-10. The clinical and research drafts of ICD-10 were thoroughly reviewed by the DSM-IV Work Groups and suggested important topics for DSM-IV literature reviews and data reanalyses. The ICD-10 diagnostic criteria for research were included as alternatives to be compared with DSM-III, DSM-III-R and suggested DSM-IV criteria sets in the DSM-IV field trials. The many consultations between the developers of DSM-IV and ICD-10 (which were facilitated by the National Institute of Mental Health, the National Institute of Drug Abuse, and the National Institute on Alcohol Abuse and Alcoholism) have been enormously useful in increasing the congruence and reducing meaningless differences in wording between the two systems.

DEFINITION OF MENTAL DISORDER

Although this volume is titled the Diagnostic and Statistical Manual of Mental Disorders, the term "mental disorder" unfortunately implies a distinction between "mental" disorders and "physical" disorders that is a reductionistic anachronism of mind/body dualism. A compelling literature documents that there is much "physical" in "mental" disorders and much "mental" in "physical" disorders. The problem raised by the term "mental" disorders has been much clearer than its solution, and, unfortunately, the term persists in the title of DSM-IV because we have not found an appropriate substitute.

Moreover, although this manual provides a classification of mental disorders, it must be admitted that no definition adequately specifies precise boundaries for the concept "mental disorder." The concept of mental disorder, like many other concepts in medicine and science, lacks a consistent operational definition that covers all situations. All medical illnesses are defined on various levels of abstraction: for example, structural pathology (e.g., ulcerative colitis), symptom presentation (e.g., migraine), deviance from a physiological norm (e.g., hypertension), and etiology (e.g., pneumococcal pneumonia). Attempts to define mental disorders have also been based on similar fallible indicators each of which may fall short when dealing with particular boundary cases.

Despite these caveats it is useful to present the definition of "mental disorder" that was included in DSM-III and DSM-III-R because it is as serviceable as any other available definition and has helped to guide decisions regarding which conditions on the border between normality and pathology should be included in DSM-IV. In DSM-IV, each of the mental disorders is conceptualized as a clinically significant behavioral or psychological syndrome or pattern that occurs in an individual and that is associated with present distress (a painful symptom) or disability (impairment in one or more important areas of functioning) or with a significantly increased risk of suffering death, pain, disability, or an important loss of freedom. In addition, this syndrome or pattern must not be merely an expectable and culturally sanctioned response to a particular event, e.g., the death of a loved one. Whatever its original cause, it must currently be considered a manifestation of a behavioral, psychological, or biological dysfunction in the individual. Neither deviant behavior, e.g., political, religious, or sexual, nor conflicts that are primarily between the individual and society are mental disorders unless the deviance or conflict is a symptom of a dysfunction in the individual, as described above.

A common misconception is that a classification of mental disorders classifies people, when actually what are being classified are disorders that people have. For this reason, the text of DSM-IV (as did the text of DSM-III-R) avoids the use of such expressions as "a schizophrenic" or "an alcoholic," and instead uses the more accurate, but admittedly more cumbersome, "a person with Schizophrenia" or "a person with Alcohol Dependence."

CAVEATS IN THE USE OF DSM-IV

Limitations of the Categorical Approach: DSM-IV is a categorical classification which divides mental disorders into types based on criteria sets with defining features. This naming of categories is the traditional method of organizing and transmitting information in everyday life and has been the fundamental approach used in all systems of medical diagnosis. A categorical approach to classification works best when all members of a diagnostic class are homogeneous, when there are clear boundaries between classes, and when the different classes are mutually exclusive. Nonetheless, the limitations of the categorical classification system must be recognized.

In DSM-IV, there is no assumption that each category of mental disorder is a completely discrete entity with absolute boundaries dividing it from other mental disorders or from no mental disorder. There is also no assumption that all people described as having the same mental disorder are alike in all important ways. The clinician using DSM-IV should therefore consider that individuals sharing a diagnosis are likely to be heterogeneous even in regard to the defining features of the diagnosis and that border cases will be difficult to diagnose in any but a probabilistic fashion. This outlook allows greater flexibility in the use of the system, encourages more specific attention to boundary cases, and emphasizes the need to capture additional clinical information that goes beyond diagnosis. In recognition of the heterogeneity of clinical presentations, DSM-IV often includes polythetic criteria sets, in which the individual need only present with a subset of items from a longer list (e.g., the diagnosis of Borderline Personality Disorder requires only five out of nine items).

It was suggested that the DSM-IV classification be organized following a dimensional model rather than the categorical model used in DSM-III-R. A dimensional system classifies clinical presentations based on quantification of attributes rather than the assignment of categories and works best in describing phenomena which are distributed continuously and do not have clear boundaries. Although dimensional systems save information and increase reliability, they also have serious limitations and thus far have been less useful than categorical systems in clinical practice and in stimulating research. Numerical dimensional descriptions are much less familiar and vivid than are the categorical names for mental disorders. Moreover, there is as yet no agreement on the choice of the optimal dimensions to be used for classification purposes. Nonetheless, it is possible that the increasing research on, and familiarity with, dimensional systems may eventually result in their greater acceptance both as a method of conveying clinical information and as a research tool.

Use of Clinical Judgment: DSM-IV is a classification of mental disorders that was developed for use in clinical, educational, and research settings. The diagnostic categories, criteria, and textual descriptions are meant to be employed by individuals with appropriate clinical training and experience in diagnosis. It is important that DSM-IV not be applied mechanically by untrained individuals. The specific diagnostic criteria included in DSM-IV are meant to serve as guidelines to be informed by clinical judgment and are not meant to be used in a cookbook fashion. For example, the exercise of clinical judgment may justify giving the diagnosis to an individual when the clinical presentation falls just short of meeting the full criteria for the diagnosis as long as the symptoms that are present are persistent and severe. On the other hand, lack of familiarity with, or excessively flexible and idiosyncratic application of DSM-IV, substantially reduces its utility as a common language for communication.

Use of DSM-IV in Forensic Settings: When the DSM-IV categories, criteria, and textual descriptions are employed for forensic purposes, there are significant risks that diagnostic information will be misused or misunderstood. These dangers arise because of the imperfect fit between the questions of ultimate concern to the law and the information contained in a clinical diagnosis. In most situations, the clinical diagnosis of a DSM-IV mental disorder is not sufficient to establish the existence for legal purposes of a "mental disorder," "mental disability," "mental disease," or "mental defect." In determining whether an individual meets a specified legal standard (e.g., for competence, criminal responsibility, or disability) additional information is usually required beyond that contained in the DSM-IV diagnosis. This might include information about the individual's functional impairments, and how these impairments affect the particular abilities in question. It is precisely because impairments, abilities, and disabilities vary widely within each diagnostic category that assignment of a particular diagnosis does not imply a specific level of impairment or disability.

Non-clinical decision makers should also be cautioned that a diagnosis does not carry any necessary implications regarding the causes of the individual's mental disorder or its associated impairments. Inclusion of a disorder in the classification (as in medicine generally) does not require that there be knowledge about its etiology. Moreover, the fact that an individual's presentation meets the criteria for a DSM-IV diagnosis does not carry any necessary implication regarding the individual's degree of control over the behaviors that may be associated with the disorder. Even when diminished control over one's behavior is a feature of the disorder, having the diagnosis in itself does not demonstrate that a particular individual is (or was) unable to control his or her behavior at a particular time.

It must be noted that DSM-IV reflects a consensus about the classification and diagnosis of mental disorders derived at the time of its initial publication. New knowledge generated by research or clinical experience will undoubtedly lead to an increased understanding of the disorders included in DSM-IV, to the identification of new disorders, and to the removal of some disorders in future classifications. The text and criteria sets included in DSM-IV will require reconsideration in light of evolving new information.

The use of DSM-IV in forensic settings should be informed by an awareness of the risks discussed above. When used appropriately, diagnoses and diagnostic information can assist decision makers in their determinations. For example, when the presence of a mental disorder is the predicate for a subsequent legal determination (e.g., involuntary civil commitment), the use of an established system of diagnosis enhances the value and reliability of the determination. By providing a compendium based upon a review of the pertinent clinical and research literature, DSM-IV may facilitate the legal decision-makers' understanding of the relevant characteristics of mental disorders. The literature related to diagnoses also serves as a check on ungrounded speculation about mental disorders and about the functioning of a particular individual. Finally, diagnostic information regarding longitudinal course may improve decision-making when the legal issue concerns an individual's mental functioning at a past or future point in time.

Use in Cross-cultural Settings: Special caution must be exercised when a clinician from one ethnic or cultural group uses the DSM-IV classification to evaluate an individual from a different ethnic or cultural group. A clinician who is unfamiliar with the nuances of an individual's cultural frame of reference may incorrectly judge as psychopathology those normal variations in behavior, belief, or experience that are particular to the individual's culture. For example, certain religious practices or beliefs (e.g., hearing or seeing a deceased relative during bereavement) may be misdiagnosed as manifestations of a psychotic disorder. Applying personality disorder criteria across cultural settings may be especially difficult because of the wide cultural variation in concepts of self, styles of communication, and coping mechanisms.

DSM-IV includes two types of information specifically related to cultural variations in mental disorders: 1) cultural variations in the clinical presentations of those disorders that have been included in the DSM-IV classification; and 2) the description of culture-bound syndromes that have not been included in the DSM-IV classification.

The wide international acceptance of the Diagnostic and Statistical Manual of Mental Disorders suggests that this classification is useful in describing mental disorders as these present in individuals throughout the world. Nonetheless, there is also evidence suggesting that the symptoms and course of a number of DSM-IV disorders are influenced by local cultural factors. In order to facilitate the application of DSM-IV to individuals from diverse cultural and ethnic settings, DSM-IV includes a new section in the text to cover culturally-related features. This section describes culturally-specific symptom patterns, preferred idioms for describing distress, and prevalence when such information is available. It will provide the clinician with guidance on how the clinical presentation may be influenced by the individual's cultural setting (e.g., depressive disorders are characterized by a preponderance of somatic symptoms rather than sadness in certain cultures.)

The second type of cultural variation pertains to "culture-bound syndromes" that have been described in just one, or a few, of the world's societies. DSM-IV provides two ways of increasing the recognition of culture-bound syndromes: 1) some (e.g., amok, ataques de nervios) are included as separate examples in Not Otherwise Specified categories; and 2) DSM-IV has also introduced an appendix of culture-bound syndromes (Appendix I) that includes the name for the condition, the cultures in which it was first described, a brief description of the psychopathology, and a list of possibly-related DSM-IV categories.

The provision of a culture-specific section in the DSM-IV text and the inclusion of a glossary of culture-bound syndromes are designed to enhance the cross-cultural applicability of DSM-IV. It is hoped that these new features will increase sensitivity to variations in how mental disorders present in different cultures and will reduce the possible effect of unintended bias stemming from the clinician's own cultural background.

Use of DSM-IV in Treatment Planning: Making a DSM-IV diagnosis is only the first step in a comprehensive evaluation. To formulate an adequate treatment plan, the clinician will invariably require considerable additional information about the person being evaluated beyond that required to make a DSM-IV diagnosis.

Distinction Between "Mental Disorder" and "General Medical Condition": The terms "mental disorder" and "general medical condition" are used throughout this manual. The term "mental disorder" is explained above. As used in this manual, it refers to the categories contained in the Mental Disorders Chapter of the ICD. The term "general medical condition" is used merely as a convenient shorthand to refer to conditions and disorders that are listed outside the Mental Disorders section of the ICD. It should be recognized that these are merely terms of convenience and should not be taken to imply that there is any fundamental distinction between mental disorders and general medical conditions, that mental disorders are unrelated to physical or biological factors or processes, or that general medical conditions are unrelated to behavioral or psychosocial factors or processes.

ORGANIZATION OF THE MANUAL

The next chapter provides instructions concerning the use of the manual. This is followed by a listing of the disorders that comprise the DSM-IV classification, which includes the ICD-9-CM code for each disorder. Next is a chapter describing the multiaxial system that can be used in reporting DSM-IV diagnoses. Then comes the main body of DSM-IV which contains a systematic presentation of the text description and diagnostic criteria set for each of the DSM-IV disorders. Finally, DSM-IV includes 10 appendices: A) Diagnostic Decision Trees; B) Criteria Sets and Axes Provided for

Further Study; C) Glossary of Technical Terms; D) Annotated Comparative Listing
Between DSM-IV/DSM-III-R; E) Numeric Listing of DSM-IV Diagnoses and Codes; F)
Alphabetic Listing of DSM-IV Diagnoses and Codes; G) Selected ICD Codes for General
Medical Conditions; H) Corresponding ICD-10 Codes for DSM-IV Disorders; I) Culturally-
Related Syndromes; J) List of DSM-IV Participants.

CAUTIONARY STATEMENT

The specified diagnostic criteria for each mental disorder are offered as guidelines for making diagnoses, since it has been demonstrated that the use of such criteria enhances agreement among clinicians and investigators. The proper use of these criteria requires specialized clinical training that provides both a body of knowledge and clinical skills.

These diagnostic criteria and the DSM-IV classification of mental disorders reflect a consensus of current formulations of evolving knowledge in our field but do not encompass all the conditions that may be legitimate focuses of treatment or research efforts.

The purpose of DSM-IV is to provide clear descriptions of diagnostic categories in order to enable clinicians and investigators to diagnose, communicate about, study, and treat the various mental disorders. It is to be understood that inclusion here, for clinical and research purposes, of a diagnostic category such as Pathological Gambling or Pedophilia does not imply that the condition meets legal or other nonmedical criteria for what constitutes mental disease, mental disorder, or mental disability. The clinical and scientific considerations involved in categorization of these conditions as mental disorders may not be wholly relevant to legal judgments, for example, that take into account such issues as individual responsibility, disability determination, and competency.

Use of the Manual

CODING AND REPORTING PROCEDURES

Diagnostic Codes

The official coding system in use as of publication of this manual is the International Classification of Diseases, Ninth Revision, Clinical Modification (ICD-9-CM). Most DSM-IV disorders have a numerical ICD-9-CM code which appears several times: 1) preceding the name of the disorder in the classification (pages xx-xx); 2) at the beginning of the text section for each disorder; and 3) accompanying the criteria set for each disorder. For some diagnoses (e.g., Mental Retardation, Substance-induced Mood Disorder), the appropriate code depends on further specification and is listed after the text and criteria set for the disorder. Most disorders have four digit codes although some have a fifth digit, usually to provide greater specificity. The names of some disorders are followed by alternative terms enclosed in parentheses which, in most cases, were the DSM-III-R names for the disorders.

The fifth digit is often used to code subtypes and modifiers of the disorder. Subtypes define a variety of mutually exclusive and jointly exhaustive subgroupings within a diagnosis and are indicated by the instruction "specify type." For example, Delusional Disorder is subtyped based on the content of the delusions, with seven subtypes provided: erotomanic type, grandiose type, jealous type, persecutory type, somatic type, mixed type, and unspecified type. If the clinician does not know which type applies or chooses not to indicate a type, the unspecified type may be used. In contrast, modifiers are not intended to be mutually exclusive or jointly exhaustive, and are indicated by the instruction "specify if" (e.g, for Social Phobia, the instruction notes "Specify if: generalized"). Modifiers provide an opportunity to define a more homogeneous subgrouping of individuals with the disorder who share certain features in common (for example, the age of onset modifier in Conduct Disorder or the syndromal feature modifier in "Major Depressive Disorder, With Melancholic Features"). Although a fifth digit is sometimes assigned to code a subtype or modifier (e.g., 290.12 Dementia of the Alzheimer's Type, Early Onset, with delusions) or severity (296.21 Major Depressive Disorder, Single Episode, Mild), the vast majority of specifiers and subtypes included in DSM-IV cannot be coded within the ICD-9-CM system and are indicated only by including the subtype or modifier after the name of the disorder (e.g., Social Phobia, Generalized).

The use of diagnostic codes is fundamental to medical record keeping. Diagnostic coding facilitates data collection and retrieval, and compiling of statistical information. Codes are also often required in the reporting of diagnostic data to interested third parties, including governmental agencies, private insurers, and the World Health Organization. For example, in the United States, the use of these codes has been mandated by the Health Care Financing Administration (HCFA) for purposes of reimbursement under the Medicare system.

Severity and Course Modifiers

A DSM-IV diagnosis is usually applied to the individual's current presentation and is not typically used to denote any previous diagnoses from which the individual has recovered. The following modifiers indicating severity and course may be listed after the diagnosis: mild, moderate, severe, in partial remission and in full remission.

The modifiers "mild," "moderate," and "severe" should be used only when the full criteria for the disorder are currently met. In deciding whether the presentation should be described as mild, moderate, or severe, the clinician should take into account the number and intensity of the signs and symptoms of the disorder and any resulting impairment in occupational or social functioning. Specific criteria for defining the mild, moderate, and severe levels of severity and partial and full remission, have been provided for the following disorders: Mental Retardation, Attention-deficit/Hyperactivity Disorder, Conduct Disorder, Oppositional Defiant Disorder, Dementia, Manic Episode, Major Depressive Episode, Paraphilias, and Substance Dependence.

For all the other disorders, the following guidelines may be used:

Mild: Few, if any, symptoms in excess of those required to make the diagnosis and symptoms result in no more than minor impairment in social or occupational functioning.

Moderate: Symptoms or functional impairment between "mild" and "severe."

Severe: Many symptoms in excess of those required to make the diagnosis, or several symptoms that are particularly severe, or the symptoms result in marked impairment in social or occupational functioning.

In Partial Remission: The full criteria for the disorder were previously met, but currently only some of the symptoms or signs of the illness remain.   This modifier may also be used when some of the symptoms or signs have reappeared following a period of full remission.

In Full Remission: There are no longer any symptoms or signs of the disorder but it is still clinically relevant to note a history of the disorder. For example, an individual with previous episodes of Bipolar Disorder who has been symptom-free on Lithium for the past three years.

After a period of time in full remission, the clinician may judge the individual to be recovered and therefore would no longer code the disorder as a current diagnosis. The differentiation of "in full remission" from "recovered" requires consideration of many factors including: the characteristic course of the disorder, the length of time since the last period of disturbance, the total duration of the disturbance, and the need for continued evaluation or prophylactic treatment.

Prior History: For some purposes, it may be useful to note a past history of having met the criteria for a disorder even when the individual is considered to be recovered from it. Such past diagnoses of mental disorder would be indicated by using the modifier "prior history" (e.g., Separation Anxiety Disorder, Prior History in an individual who has no current disorder or who currently meets criteria for Panic Disorder).

Principal Diagnosis

When more than one diagnosis is given, the principal diagnosis is the condition established after study to be chiefly responsible for occasioning the admission of the patient to clinical care. In most cases, it is also the main focus of attention or treatment. It is often difficult (and somewhat arbitrary) to determine which diagnosis is the principal diagnosis, especially in situations of "dual diagnosis" (a substance use diagnosis like Amphetamine Dependence accompanied by a non-substance use diagnosis like Schizophrenia). For example, it may be unclear which diagnosis should be considered "principal" for an individual hospitalized with both Schizophrenia and Amphetamine Intoxication, since each condition may have contributed equally to the need for admission and treatment.

Multiple diagnoses can be reported in a multiaxial fashion (see page xx) or in a nonaxial fashion (see page xx). When the principal diagnosis is an Axis I disorder, this is indicated by listing it first. The remaining disorders are listed in order of focus of attention and treatment. When a person has both an Axis I and an Axis II diagnosis, the principal diagnosis will be assumed to be on Axis I unless the Axis II diagnosis is followed by the qualifying phrase "(Principal diagnosis)."

Provisional diagnosis

The modifier "provisional" can be used when there is a strong presumption that the full criteria will be met for a disorder, but not enough information is available to make a firm diagnosis. The clinician can indicate the diagnostic uncertainty by writing "(Provisional)" following the diagnosis. For example, the individual appears to have a Major Depressive Disorder but is unable to give an adequate history to establish that the full criteria are met. Another use of the term "provisional" is for those situations in which differential diagnosis depends exclusively on the duration of illness. For example, a diagnosis of Schizophreniform Disorder requires a duration of less than six months and can only be given provisionally if assigned before remission has occurred.

Use of Not Otherwise Specified Categories

Because of the diversity of clinical presentations, it is impossible for the diagnostic nomenclature to cover every possible situation. For this reason, each diagnostic class has at least one Not Otherwise Specified (NOS) category and some classes have several NOS categories. There are four situations in which the NOS diagnosis may be appropriate: 1) The presentation conforms to the general guidelines for a mental disorder in the diagnostic class or subgrouping, but the symptomatic picture does not meet the criteria for any of the specific disorders. This would occur either when the symptoms are below the diagnostic threshold for one of the specific disorders or if there is an atypical or mixed presentation; 2) The presentation conforms to a disorder that has not been included in the DSM-IV classification. Some of these disorders have been included in Appendix B (for Criteria Sets and Axes Provided for Further Study) in which case a page reference to the suggested criteria sets is provided; 3) NOS can be used when there is uncertainty about etiology (i.e., whether the disorder is due to a general medical condition, is substance-induced, or is primary); 4) NOS can be used when there is insufficient opportunity for complete data collection (e.g., emergency situations), or inconsistent or contradictory information, but there is enough information to place it within a particular diagnostic class (e.g., the clinician determines the individual has psychotic symptoms but does not have enough information to diagnose a specific Psychotic Disorder).

Ways of Indicating Diagnostic Uncertainty

The following table indicates the various ways in which a clinician may indicate diagnostic uncertainty:

Term	Examples of clinical situations
V Codes (for Other Conditions That May Be a Focus of Clinical Attention)	Insufficient information to know whether or not a presenting problem is attributa to a mental disorder, e.g., Academic Problem; Adult Antisocial Behavior.
799.90 Diagnosis or Condition Deferred on Axis I	Information inadequate to make any diagnostic judgment about an Axis I diagnosis or condition.
799.90 Diagnosis Deferred on Axis II	Same for an Axis II diagnosis.
300.90 Unspecified Mental Disorder (nonpsychotic)	Enough information available to rule out a psychotic disorder, but further specification is not possible.
298.90 Psychotic Disorder Not Otherwise Specified	Enough information available to determi the presence of a psychotic disorder, b further specification is not possible.
(Class of disorder) Not Otherwise Specified	Enough information available to indicat the class of disorder that is present,

but further specification is not possible, because either there is not sufficient information to make a more specific diagnosis, or the clinical features of the disorder do not meet the criteria for any of the specific categories in that class, e.g., Depressive Disorder Not Otherwise Specified.

Specific diagnosis (Provisional)   Enough information available to make a "working" diagnosis, but the clinician wishes to indicate a significant degree of diagnostic uncertainty, e.g., Schizophreniform Disorder (Provisional)

FREQUENTLY USED CRITERIA

Criteria to Exclude Other Diagnoses and to Suggest Differential Diagnoses

Most of the criteria sets presented in this manual include exclusion criteria that are necessary to establish boundaries between disorders and to clarify differential diagnoses. The several different wordings of exclusion criteria in the criteria sets throughout DSM-IV reflect the different types of possible relationships between disorders:

1) **"has never met the criteria for..."** This exclusion criterion is used to define a lifetime hierarchy between disorders, (e.g., a diagnosis of Major Depressive Disorder can no longer be given once a manic episode has occurred and must be changed to a diagnosis of Bipolar Disorder).

2) **"does not meet the criteria for..."** This exclusion criterion is used to establish a hierarchy between disorders (or subtypes) defined cross-sectionally (e.g., a diagnosis of Schizoaffective Disorder excludes a simultaneous diagnosis of Schizophrenia; The "with melancholic features" modifier takes precedence over the "with atypical features" modifier for describing the current major depressive episode).

3) **"does not occur exclusively during the course of..."** This exclusion criterion prevents a disorder from being diagnosed when its symptom presentation occurs only during the course of another disorder (e.g., Dementia is not diagnosed separately if it occurs only during Delirium; Conversion Disorder is not diagnosed separately if it occurs only during Somatization Disorder; Bulimia Nervosa is not diagnosed separately if it occurs only during Anorexia Nervosa). This exclusion criterion is typically used in situations in which the symptoms of one disorder are associated features or a subset of the symptoms of the preempting disorder. It should be noted that the excluded diagnosis can be given at times when it occurs independently.

4) **"not due to the direct effects of a substance (e.g., drugs of abuse, medication) or a general medical condition."** This exclusion is used to indicate that a substance-induced and general medical etiology must be considered and ruled out before the

disorder can be diagnosed (e.g., Major Depressive Disorder can only be diagnosed once etiologies based on substance use and medical illness have been ruled out).

5) **"not better accounted for by..."** This exclusion criterion is used to indicate that the disorders mentioned in the criterion must be considered in the differential diagnosis of the presenting psychopathology and that, in boundary cases, clinical judgment will be necessary in order to determine which disorder provides the most appropriate diagnosis. In such cases, the differential diagnosis section of the text should be consulted for guidance.

The general convention in DSM-IV allows multiple diagnoses to be assigned for those individuals who meet criteria for more than one DSM-IV disorder. There are three situations in which the above mentioned exclusion criteria are included within the criteria sets in order to establish a diagnostic hierarchy (and thus to prevent multiple diagnoses) or to highlight differential diagnostic considerations (and thus to discourage multiple diagnoses):

1) When a Mental Disorder Due to a General Medical Condition or a Substance-induced Disorder is responsible for the symptoms, it preempts the diagnosis of any other disorder with the same symptoms (e.g., Cocaine Mood Disorder preempts Major Depressive Disorder). In such cases, an exclusion criterion containing the phrase "not due to the direct effects of..." is included.

2) When a more pervasive disorder has among its defining symptoms (or associated symptoms) what are the defining symptoms of a less pervasive disorder, one of the following three exclusion criteria indicates that only the more pervasive disorder is diagnosed: "has never met the criteria for...", "does not meet the criteria for...", "does not occur exclusively during the course of...". For example, Schizophrenia may have chronic depression (a defining feature of Dysthymic Disorder) as an associated feature. Because Schizophrenia is more pervasive than Dysthymic Disorder, an exclusion criterion is included in Dysthymic Disorder that prevents its diagnosis if it occurs only during the course of Schizophrenia..

3) When there are particularly difficult differential diagnostic boundaries, the phrase "not better accounted for by..." is included to indicate that clinical judgment is necessary to determine which diagnosis is most appropriate (e.g., Panic Disorder with Agoraphobia includes the criterion "not better accounted for by Social Phobia" and Social Phobia includes the criterion "not better accounted for by Panic Disorder with Agoraphobia" in recognition of the fact that this is a particularly difficult boundary to draw).

Criteria for Substance-Induced Disorders

The relationship between substance use and presenting symptomatology is a crucial, but inherently difficult, clinical determination. In an effort to provide some assistance, the two criteria listed below have been added to each of the substance-induced disorders. These criteria are intended to provide general guidelines, but at the same time allow for clinical judgment in determining whether or not the presenting symptoms are best accounted for by use of the substance. For further discussion of this issue, see page xx.

B. There is evidence from the history, physical examination, or laboratory findings of substance intoxication or withdrawal, and the symptoms developed during, or within a month of, significant substance intoxication or withdrawal.

C. The disturbance is not better accounted for by a disorder that is not substance-induced. Evidence that the symptoms are better accounted for by a disorder that is not substance-induced might include: the symptoms precede the onset of the substance abuse or dependence; persist for a substantial period of time (e.g., about a month) after the cessation of acute withdrawal or severe intoxication; are substantially in excess of what would be expected given the character, duration, or amount of the substance used; or there is other evidence suggesting the existence of an independent non-substance-induced disorder (e.g., a history of recurrent non-substance-related episodes).

Criteria for a Mental Disorder Due to a General Medical Condition

The criterion listed below is necessary to establish the etiologic requirement for each of the Mental Disorders Due to a General Medical Condition (e.g., Mood Disorder Due to Hypothyroidism). For further discussion of this issue, see page xx.

There is evidence from the history, physical examination, or laboratory findings of a general medical condition judged to be etiologically related to the disturbance.

Criteria for Clinical Significance

The definition of "mental disorder" in the introduction to DSM-IV requires that there be clinically significant impairment or distress as an inherent feature of the disorders in the nomenclature. In order to highlight the importance of considering this issue, the criteria sets for a number of disorders include a clinical significance criterion (usually worded "...causes clinically significant distress or impairment in social, occupational, or other important areas of functioning"). This helps establish the threshold for the diagnosis of a disorder in those situations in which the symptomatic presentation by itself (particularly in its milder forms) is not inherently pathological and may be encountered in individuals for which a diagnosis of "mental disorder" would be inappropriate.

TYPES OF INFORMATION IN THE DSM-IV TEXT

The text of DSM-IV systematically describes each disorder under the following headings: diagnostic features; associated features and disorders; specific age, cultural, or gender-related features; prevalence, incidence, and risk; course; complications; predisposing factors; familial pattern; and differential diagnosis. In some instances, when many of the specific disorders share common features, this information is included in the introduction to the entire section.

<u>Diagnostic Features</u>: This section clarifies the diagnostic criteria and often provides illustrative examples.

<u>Associated Features and Disorders</u>: This section is subdivided into three parts:
1) Associated Descriptive Features and Mental Disorders: This includes clinical features that are frequently associated with the disorder but are not considered essential to making the diagnosis. In some cases, these features were considered for inclusion as possible diagnostic criteria but were insufficiently sensitive or specific to be included in the final criteria set. Also noted in this section are other mental disorders associated with the disorder being discussed. It is specified (when known) if these disorders precede, co-occur with, or are consequences of the disorder in question (for example, alcohol-induced dementia is a consequence of chronic alcohol dependence).

2) Associated Laboratory Findings: This section provides information on three types of laboratory findings associated with the disorder: a) Those associated laboratory findings that have sufficient sensitivity and specificity to be considered "diagnostic" of the disorder, for example, polysomnographic findings in certain sleep disorders; b) Those associated laboratory findings that are confirmatory of the construct of the disorder but that do not have sufficiently documented sensitivity and specificity to be useful in the diagnosis of a given individual, for example, ventricle size on CT scan as validator of the construct of Schizophrenia; c) Those laboratory findings that are associated with the complications of a disorder, for example, electrolyte imbalances in individuals with Anorexia Nervosa.

3) Associated Physical Examination Signs, Symptoms, and General Medical Conditions: This section includes symptoms elicited by history, or signs noted during physical examination, which may be of diagnostic significance but are not essential to the diagnosis, e.g., dental erosion in Bulimia Nervosa. Also included are those disorders coded outside the Mental Disorders section of ICD that are associated with the disorder being discussed. As is done for associated mental disorders, the type of association (i.e., precedes, co-occurs with, is a consequence of) is specified if known. For example, cirrhosis is a consequence of Alcohol Dependence.

<u>Specific Age-Related or Culturally-Related or Gender-Related Features</u>: This section provides guidance for the clinician concerning variations in the presentation of the disorder that may be attributable to the individual's developmental stage (e.g., infancy, childhood, adolescence, late life), cultural setting, or gender. This section also includes information on differential prevalence rates (e.g., sex ratio).

<u>Prevalence, Incidence, and Risk</u>: This section provides data on point and lifetime prevalence, incidence and lifetime risk. These data are provided for different settings (e.g., community, outpatient, and inpatient) when this information is known.

<u>Course:</u> This section describes the typical lifetime patterns of presentation and evolution of the disorder and is divided into four subsections: 1) typical **age at onset** and **mode of onset** (e.g., abrupt or insidious) of the disorder and 2) **single episode** vs. **recurrent,**

episodic vs. **continuous course** referring to whether there are distinct periods of illness separated by intervals free of symptoms; 3) **duration** characterizing the typical length of the illness and its episodes; 4) **progression** describing the general trend of the disorder over time (e.g., stationary, worsening, improving)

Complications: This describes the types of serious morbidity that may occur as a result of the disorder (e.g., suicide, divorce, homelessness, violence, incarceration, school suspension, unemployment, loss of job, etc.).

Familial Pattern: This describes data on the frequency of the disorder among first-degree biologic relatives of those with the disorder compared with the frequency in the general population. It also indicates other disorders that tend to occur more frequently in family members of those with the disorder.

Differential Diagnosis: This section discusses how to differentiate this disorder from those other disorders that have some similar presenting characteristics.

Predisposing Factors: This section describes characteristics of a person that can be identified before the development of the disorder and place the person at a higher risk for developing the disorder.

DSM-IV ORGANIZATIONAL PLAN

The DSM-IV disorders are grouped into 16 major diagnostic classes (e.g., Substance-related Disorders, Mood Disorders, Anxiety Disorders, etc.) and one additional section for Other Conditions That May Be a Focus of Clinical Attention. The manual begins with the DSM-IV Classification (pages xx-xx) which provides a systematic listing of the official codes and categories. Next is a description of the DSM-IV Multiaxial System for diagnosis (pages xx-xx). This is followed by the diagnostic criteria for each of the DSM-IV disorders accompanied by descriptive text (pages xx-xx).

The first section is devoted to Disorders Usually First Diagnosed in Infancy, Childhood, or Adolescence. This division of the classification according to age of presentation is for general convenience only and is not absolute. While disorders in this section are "usually first evident in childhood and adolescence," some individuals diagnosed with disorders located in this section may not present for clinical attention until adulthood. In addition, the age of onset for many disorders placed in other sections is not uncommonly during childhood or adolescence (e.g., Major Depressive Disorder, Schizophrenia, Generalized Anxiety Disorder). Clinicians who work primarily with children and adolescents should therefore be familiar with the entire manual, while those who work primarily with adults should also be familiar with this section.

The next three sections (i.e., Delirium, Dementia, Amnestic and Other Cognitive Disorders; Mental Disorders Due to a General Medical Condition, and Substance-Related Disorders) were grouped together in DSM-III-R under the single heading of "Organic Mental Disorders." The term "organic mental disorder" is no longer used in DSM-IV because it incorrectly implies that the other mental disorders in the manual do not have a biologic basis. As in DSM-III-R, these sections are placed before the remaining disorders in the manual because of their priority in differential diagnosis (e.g., substance-related causes of depressed mood must be ruled out before making a diagnosis of Major Depressive Disorder). In order to facilitate differential diagnosis, complete lists of Mental Disorders Due to a General Medical Condition and Substance-Related disorders appear in these sections, while the text and criteria for these disorders are placed in the diagnostic section with which they share phenomenology. For example, the text and criteria for Substance-induced Mood Disorder and Mood Disorder Due to a General Medical Condition are included in the Mood Disorders section.

The organizing principle for all the remaining sections (except for Adjustment Disorders) is to group together disorders based on their shared phenomenologic features in order to facilitate differential diagnosis.

The Adjustment Disorders section is organized differently in that these disorders are grouped together based on their common etiology (e.g., maladaptive reaction to a stressor). Therefore, the Adjustment Disorders include a variety of heterogeneous clinical presentations (e.g., Adjustment Disorder With Depressed Mood, Adjustment Disorder With Anxiety, Adjustment Disorder With Disturbance of Conduct).

Finally DSM-IV includes a section for Other Conditions That May be a Focus of Clinical Attention.

DSM-IV Classification

Note: These codes are preliminary and are subject to further updates and modifications after additional consultations.

DISORDERS USUALLY FIRST DIAGNOSED IN INFANCY, CHILDHOOD, OR ADOLESCENCE

Mental Retardation
- 317   Mild Mental Retardation
- 318.0   Moderate Retardation
- 318.1   Severe Mental Retardation
- 318.2   Profound Mental Retardation
- 319   Mental Retardation, Severity Unspecified

Learning Disorders (Academic Skills Disorder)
- 315.00   Reading Disorder (Developmental Reading Disorder)
- 315.1   Mathematics Disorder (Developmental Arithmetic Disorder)
- 315.2   Disorder of Written Expression (Developmental Expressive Writing Disorder)
- 315.9   Learning Disorder NOS

Motor Skills Disorder
- 315.4   Developmental Coordination Disorder

Pervasive Developmental Disorders
- 299.00   Autistic Disorder
- 299.80   Rett's Disorder
- 299.10   Childhood Disintegrative Disorder
  - Asperger's Disorder (? placement)
- 299.80   Pervasive Developmental Disorder NOS (including Atypical Autism)

Disruptive Behavior and Attention-deficit Disorders

         Attention-deficit/Hyperactivity Disorder
- 314.00   predominantly inattentive type
- 314.01   predominantly hyperactive-impulsive type
- 314.01   combined type
- 314.9   Attention-deficit/Hyperactivity Disorder NOS
- 313.81   Oppositional Defiant Disorder
- 312.8   Conduct Disorder
- 312.9   Disruptive Behavior Disorder NOS

Feeding and Eating Disorders of Infancy or Early Childhood
    307.52   Pica
    307.53   Rumination Disorder
    307.59   Feeding Disorder of Infancy or Early Childhood

Tic Disorders
    307.23   Tourette's Disorder
    307.22   Chronic Motor or Vocal Tic Disorder
    307.21   Transient Tic Disorder
    307.20   Tic Disorder NOS

Communication Disorders
    315.31   Expressive Language Disorder (Developmental Expressive Language Disorder)
    315.31   Mixed Receptive/Expressive Language Disorder (Developmental Receptive Language Disorder)
    315.39   Phonological Disorder (Developmental Articulation Disorder)
    307.0   Stuttering
    315.39   Communication Disorder NOS

Elimination Disorders
    307.7   Encopresis
    307.6   Enuresis

Other Disorders of Infancy, Childhood, or Adolescence
    309.21   Separation Anxiety Disorder
    313.23   Selective Mutism (Elective Mutism)
    313.89   Reactive Attachment Disorder of Infancy or Early Childhood
    307.3   Stereotypic Movement Disorder (Stereotypy/Habit Disorder)
    313.9   Disorder of Infancy, Childhood, or Adolescence NOS

DELIRIUM, DEMENTIA, AMNESTIC AND OTHER COGNITIVE DISORDERS

Deliria
    293.0   Delirium Due to a General Medical Condition
    ---.-   Substance-induced Delirium
            (refer to specific substance for code)
    ---.-   Delirium Due to Multiple Etiologies
            (use multiple codes based on specific etiologies)
    293.89   Delirium NOS

Dementias

\---.-   **Dementia of the Alzheimer's Type**
With Early Onset: if onset at age 65 or below.
       290.10 uncomplicated
       290.11 with delirium
       290.12 with delusions
       290.13 with depressed mood
       290.14 with hallucinations
       290.15 with perceptual disturbance
       290.16 with behavioral disturbance
       290.17 with communication disturbance
With Late Onset: if onset after age 65.
       290.00 uncomplicated
       290.30 with delirium
       290.20 with delusions
       290.21 with depressed mood
       290.22 with hallucinations
       290.23 with perceptual disturbance
       290.24 with behavioral disturbance
       290.25 with communication disturbance

\---.-   **Vascular Dementia (D:9)**
       290.40 uncomplicated
       290.41 with delirium
       290.42 with delusions
       290.43 with depressed mood
       290.44 with hallucinations
       290.45 with perceptual disturbance
       290.46 with behavioral disturbance
       290.47 with communication disturbance

Dementias Due to Other General Medical Conditions

294.9	**Dementia Due to HIV Disease** *(Code 043.1 on Axis III)*
294.1	**Dementia Due to Head Trauma** *(Code 905.0 on Axis III)*
294.1	**Dementia Due to Parkinson's Disease** *(Code 332.0 on Axis III)*
294.1	**Dementia Due to Huntington's Disease** *(Code 333.4 on Axis III)*
290.10	**Dementia Due to Pick's Disease** *(Code 331.1 on Axis III)*
290.10	**Dementia Due to Creutzfeldt-Jakob Disease** *(Code 046.1 on Axis III)*
294.1	**Dementia Due to Other General Medical Condition**

\---.-   **Substance-induced Persisting Dementia**
(refer to specific substance for code)

\---.-   **Dementia Due to Multiple Etiologies**
(use multiple codes based on specific etiologies)

294.8   **Dementia NOS**

Amnestic Disorders
| | |
294.0   **Amnestic Disorder Due to a General Medical Condition**
---.-   **Substance-induced Persisting Amnestic Disorder**
      (refer to specific substance for code)
294.8   **Amnestic Disorder NOS**

294.9   **Cognitive Disorder NOS**

MENTAL DISORDERS DUE TO A GENERAL MEDICAL CONDITION NOT ELSEWHERE CLASSIFIED

293.89   **Catatonic Disorder Due to a General Medical Condition**
310.1   **Personality Change Due to a General Medical Condition**
293.9   **Mental Disorder NOS Due to a General Medical Condition**

SUBSTANCE RELATED DISORDERS

Alcohol Use Disorders
303.90   **Alcohol Dependence**
305.00   **Alcohol Abuse**
303.00   **Alcohol Intoxication**
291.8   **Alcohol Withdrawal**
291.0   **Alcohol Delirium**
291.2   **Alcohol Persisting Dementia**
291.1   **Alcohol Persisting Amnestic Disorder**
      Alcohol Psychotic Disorder
291.5   **with delusions**
291.3   **with hallucinations**
291.8   **Alcohol Mood Disorder**
291.8   **Alcohol Anxiety Disorder**
292.8   **Alcohol Sexual Dysfunction**
292.89   **Alcohol Sleep Disorder**
291.9   **Alcohol Use Disorder NOS**

Amphetamine (or Related Substance) Use Disorders
304.40   **Amphetamine (or Related Substance) Dependence**
305.70   **Amphetamine (or Related Substance) Abuse**
305.70   **Amphetamine (or Related Substance) Intoxication**
292.0   **Amphetamine (or Related Substance) Withdrawal**
292.81   **Amphetamine (or Related Substance) Delirium**
      Amphetamine (or Related Substance) Psychotic Disorder
291.11   **with delusions**
291.12   **with hallucinations**
292.84   **Amphetamine (or Related Substance) Mood Disorder**
292.89   **Amphetamine (or Related Substance) Anxiety Disorder**
292.89   **Amphetamine (or Related Substance) Sexual Dysfunction**
292.89   **Amphetamine (or Related Substance) Sleep Disorder**

292.9   **Amphetamine (or Related Substance) Use Disorder NOS**

Caffeine Use Disorders

305.90   **Caffeine Intoxication**
292.84   **Caffeine Anxiety Disorder**
292.89   **Caffeine Sleep Disorder**
292.9   **Caffeine Use Disorder NOS**

Cannabis Use Disorders

304.30   **Cannabis Dependence**
305.20   **Cannabis Abuse**
305.20   **Cannabis Intoxication**
292.81   **Cannabis Delirium**
              Cannabis Psychotic Disorder
291.11   **with delusions**
291.12   **with hallucinations**
292.89   **Cannabis Anxiety Disorder**
292.9   **Cannabis Use Disorder NOS**

Cocaine Use Disorders

304.20   **Cocaine Dependence**
305.60   **Cocaine Abuse**
305.60   **Cocaine Intoxication**
292.0   **Cocaine Withdrawal**
292.81   **Cocaine Delirium**
              Cocaine Psychotic Disorder
291.11   **with delusions**
291.12   **with hallucinations**
292.84   **Cocaine Mood Disorder**
292.89   **Cocaine Anxiety Disorder**
292.89   **Cocaine Sexual Dysfunction**
292.89   **Cocaine Sleep Disorder**
292.9   **Cocaine Use Disorder NOS**

Hallucinogen Use Disorders

304.50   **Hallucinogen Dependence**
305.30   **Hallucinogen Abuse**
305.30   **Hallucinogen Intoxication**
292.89   **Hallucinogen Persisting Perception Disorder**
292.81   **Hallucinogen Delirium**
              Hallucinogen Psychotic Disorder
291.11   **with delusions**
291.12   **with hallucinations**
292.84   **Hallucinogen Mood Disorder**
292.89   **Hallucinogen Anxiety Disorder**
292.9   **Hallucinogen Use Disorder NOS**

Inhalant Use Disorders
304.60	Inhalant Dependence
305.90	Inhalant Abuse
305.90	Inhalant Intoxication
292.81	Inhalant Delirium
292.82	Inhalant Persisting Dementia
	Inhalant Psychotic Disorder
291.11	with delusions
291.12	with hallucinations
292.84	Inhalant Mood Disorder
292.89	Inhalant Anxiety Disorder
292.9	Inhalant Use Disorder NOS

Nicotine Use Disorders
305.10	Nicotine Dependence
292.0	Nicotine Withdrawal
292.9	Nicotine Use Disorder NOS

Opioid Use Disorders
304.00	Opioid Dependence
305.50	Opioid Abuse
305.50	Opioid Intoxication
292.0	Opioid Withdrawal
292.81	Opioid Delirium
	Opioid Psychotic Disorder
291.11	with delusions
291.12	with hallucinations
292.84	Opioid Mood Disorder
292.89	Opioid Sleep Disorder
292.89	Opioid Sexual Dysfunction
292.9	Opioid Use Disorder NOS

Phencyclidine (or Related Substance) Use Disorders
304.90	Phencyclidine (or Related Substance) Dependence
305.90	Phencyclidine (or Related Substance) Abuse
305.90	Phencyclidine (or Related Substance) Intoxication
292.81	Phencyclidine (or Related Substance) Delirium
	Phencyclidine (or Related Substance) Psychotic Disorder
291.11	with delusions
291.12	with hallucinations
292.84	Phencyclidine (or Related Substance) Mood Disorder
292.89	Phencyclidine (or Related Substance) Anxiety Disorder
292.9	Phencyclidine (or Related Substance) Use Disorder NOS

Sedative, Hypnotic, or Anxiolytic Substance Use Disorders
304.10   Sedative, Hypnotic, or Anxiolytic Dependence
305.40   Sedative, Hypnotic, or Anxiolytic Abuse
305.40   Sedative, Hypnotic, or Anxiolytic Intoxication
292.0   Sedative, Hypnotic, or Anxiolytic Withdrawal
292.81   Sedative, Hypnotic, or Anxiolytic Delirium
292.82   Sedative, Hypnotic, or Anxiolytic Persisting Dementia
292.83   Sedative, Hypnotic, or Anxiolytic Persisting Amnestic Disorder
  Sedative, Hypnotic, or Anxiolytic Psychotic Disorder
291.11   with delusions
291.12   with hallucinations
292.84   Sedative, Hypnotic, or Anxiolytic Mood Disorder
292.89   Sedative, Hypnotic, or Anxiolytic Anxiety Disorder
292.89   Sedative, Hypnotic, or Anxiolytic Sleep Disorder
292.89   Sedative, Hypnotic, or Anxiolytic Sexual Dysfunction
292.9   Sedative, Hypnotic, or Anxiolytic Use Disorder NOS

Polysubstance Use Disorder
304.80   Polysubstance Dependence (E:27)

Other (or Unknown) Substance Use Disorders
304.90   Other (or Unknown) Substance Dependence
305.90   Other (or Unknown) Substance Abuse
305.90   Other (or Unknown) Substance Intoxication
292.0   Other (or Unknown) Substance Withdrawal
292.81   Other (or Unknown) Substance Delirium
292.82   Other (or Unknown) Substance Persisting Dementia
292.83   Other (or Unknown) Substance Persisting Amnestic Disorder
  Other (or Unknown) Substance Psychotic Disorder
291.11   with delusions
291.12   with hallucinations
292.84   Other (or Unknown) Substance Mood Disorder
292.89   Other (or Unknown) Substance Anxiety Disorder
292.89   Other (or Unknown) Substance) Sexual Dysfunction
292.89   Other (or Unknown) Substance Sleep Disorder
292.9   Other (or Unknown) Substance Use Disorder NOS

SCHIZOPHRENIA AND OTHER PSYCHOTIC DISORDERS

Schizophrenia
295.30   paranoid type
295.10   disorganized type
295.20   catatonic type
295.90   undifferentiated type
295.60   residual type
295.40   Schizophreniform Disorder
295.70   Schizoaffective Disorder

297.1	**Delusional Disorder**
298.8	**Brief Psychotic Disorder**
297.3	**Shared Psychotic Disorder (Folie a Deux)**

Psychotic Disorder Due to a General Medical Condition

293.81	**with delusions**
293.82	**with hallucinations**
---.--	**Substance-Induced Psychotic Disorder**
	(refer to specific substances for codes)
298.9	**Psychotic Disorder NOS**

MOOD DISORDERS

Code current state of Major Depressive Disorder or Bipolar Disorder in fifth digit:

0 unspecified
1 mild
2 moderate
3 severe, without psychotic features
4 severe, with psychotic features
5 in partial remission
6 in full remission

Depressive Disorders

	Major Depressive Disorder
296.2x	**single episode**
296.3x	**recurrent**
300.4	**Dysthymic Disorder**
311	**Depressive Disorder NOS**

Bipolar Disorders

	Bipolar I Disorder
296.0x	**single manic episode**
296.4	**most recent episode hypomanic**
296.4x	**most recent episode manic**
296.6x	**most recent episode mixed**
296.5x	**most recent episode depressed**
296.7	**most recent episode unspecified**
296.89	**Bipolar II Disorder (Recurrent major depressive episodes with hypomania)**
301.13	**Cyclothymic Disorder**
296.80	**Bipolar Disorder NOS**

293.83	**Mood Disorder Due to a General Medical Condition**
---.--	**Substance-Induced Mood Disorder**
	(refer to specific substances for codes)
296.90	**Mood Disorder NOS**

ANXIETY DISORDERS

Panic Disorder
300.01	Without Agoraphobia
300.21	With Agoraphobia
300.22	Agoraphobia Without History of Panic Disorder
300.29	Specific Phobia (Simple Phobia)
300.23	Social Phobia (Social Anxiety Disorder)
300.3	Obsessive-Compulsive Disorder
309.81	Posttraumatic Stress Disorder
300.3	Acute Stress Disorder
300.02	Generalized Anxiety Disorder (includes Overanxious Disorder of Childhood)
293.89	Anxiety Disorder Due to a General Medical Condition
---.--	Substance-induced Anxiety Disorder (refer to specific substances for codes)
300.00	Anxiety Disorder NOS

SOMATOFORM DISORDERS

300.81	Somatization Disorder
300.11	Conversion Disorder
300.7	Hypochondriasis
300.71	Body Dysmorphic Disorder
	Pain Disorder
307.80	Associated with Psychological Factors
307.89	Associated with Both Psychological Factors and a General Medical Condition
300.82	Undifferentiated Somatoform Disorder
300.89	Somatoform Disorder NOS

FACTITIOUS DISORDERS

	Factitious Disorder
300.16	with predominantly psychological signs and symptoms
300.17	with predominantly physical signs and symptoms
300.18	with combined psychological and physical signs and symptoms
300.19	Factitious Disorder NOS

DISSOCIATIVE DISORDERS

300.12   Dissociative Amnesia
300.13   Dissociative Fugue
300.14   Dissociative Identity Disorder (Multiple Personality Disorder)
300.6   Depersonalization Disorder
300.15   Dissociative Disorder NOS

SEXUAL AND GENDER IDENTITY DISORDERS

Sexual Dysfunctions

Sexual Desire Disorders
302.71   Hypoactive Sexual Desire Disorder
?302.79 Sexual Aversion Disorder
Sexual Arousal Disorders
302.72   Female Sexual Arousal Disorder
302.72   Male Erectile Disorder
Orgasm Disorders
302.73   Female Orgasmic Disorder (Inhibited Female Orgasm)
302.74   Male Orgasmic Disorder (Inhibited Male Orgasm)
302.75   Premature Ejaculation
Sexual Pain Disorders
302.76   Dyspareunia
306.51   Vaginismus

Sexual Dysfunctions Due to a General Medical Condition
607.84   Male Erectile Disorder Due to a General Medical Condition
608.89   Male Dyspareunia Due to a General Medical Condition
625.0   Female Dyspareunia Due to a General Medical Condition
608.89   Male Hypoactive Sexual Desire Disorder Due to a General Medical Condition
625.8   Female Hypoactive Sexual Desire Disorder Due to a General Medical Condition
608.89   Other Male Sexual Dysfunction Due to a General Medical Condition
625.8   Other Female Sexual Dysfunction Due to a General Medical Condition
---.--   Substance-induced Sexual Dysfunction
         (refer to specific substances for codes)
302.70   Sexual Dysfunction NOS

Paraphilias

302.4	Exhibitionism
302.81	Fetishism
?302.85	Frotteurism
302.2	Pedophilia
302.83	Sexual Masochism
302.84	Sexual Sadism
302.82	Voyeurism
302.3	Transvestic Fetishism
302.9	Paraphilia NOS

302.9 Sexual Disorder NOS

Gender Identity Disorders

	Gender Identity Disorder
302.6	in Children
302.85	in Adolescents and Adults
302.6	Gender Identity Disorder NOS

EATING DISORDERS

307.1	Anorexia Nervosa
307.51	Bulimia Nervosa
307.50	Eating Disorder NOS

SLEEP DISORDERS

Primary Sleep Disorders
  Dyssomnias

307.42	Primary Insomnia
307.44	Primary Hypersomnia
347	Narcolepsy
780.59	Breathing-Related Sleep Disorder
307.45	Circadian Rhythm Sleep Disorder (Sleep-Wake Schedule Disorder)
307.47	Dyssomnia NOS

  Parasomnias

307.47	Nightmare Disorder (Dream Anxiety Disorder)
307.46	Sleep Terror Disorder
307.46	Sleepwalking Disorder
?307.47	Parasomnia NOS

Sleep Disorders Related to Another Mental Disorder

307.42	Insomnia related to [Axis I or Axis II Disorder]
307.44	Hypersomnia related to [Axis I or Axis II Disorder]

Other Sleep Disorders
    Sleep Disorder Due to a General Medical Condition
780.52   **insomnia type**
780.54   **hypersomnia type**
780.59   **parasomnia type**
780.59   **mixed type**
---.--   **Substance-Induced Sleep Disorder**
    (refer to specific substances for codes)

IMPULSE CONTROL DISORDERS NOT ELSEWHERE CLASSIFIED

312.34   **Intermittent Explosive Disorder**
312.32   **Kleptomania**
312.33   **Pyromania**
312.31   **Pathological Gambling**
?312.39   **Trichotillomania**
312.30   **Impulse Control NOS**

ADJUSTMENT DISORDERS

    Adjustment Disorder
309.24   **With Anxiety**
309.0   **With Depressed Mood**
309.3   **With Disturbance of Conduct**
309.4   **With Mixed Disturbance of Emotions and Conduct**
309.28   **With Mixed Anxiety and Depressed Mood**
309.9   **Unspecified**

PERSONALITY DISORDERS

301.0   **Paranoid Personality Disorder**
301.20   **Schizoid Personality Disorder**
301.22   **Schizotypal Personality Disorder**
301.7   **Antisocial Personality Disorder**
301.83   **Borderline Personality Disorder**
301.50   **Histrionic Personality Disorder**
301.81   **Narcissistic Personality Disorder**
301.82   **Avoidant Personality Disorder**
301.6   **Dependent Personality Disorder**
301.4   **Obsessive-Compulsive Personality Disorder**
301.9   **Personality Disorder NOS**

OTHER CONDITIONS THAT MAY BE A FOCUS OF CLINICAL ATTENTION

316 **(Psychological Factors) Affecting Medical Condition**
Choose name based on nature of factors:
Mental Disorder Affecting Medical Condition
Psychological Symptoms Affecting Medical Condition
Personality Traits or Coping Style Affecting Medical Condition
Maladaptive Health Behaviors Affecting Medical Condition
Unspecified Psychological Factors Affecting Medical Condition

Medication-Induced Movement Disorders
332.1 **Neuroleptic-induced Parkinsonism**
333.92 **Neuroleptic Malignant Syndrome**
333.7 **Neuroleptic-induced Acute Dystonia**
333.99 **Neuroleptic-induced Acute Akathisia**
333.82 **Neuroleptic-induced Tardive Dyskinesia**
333.1 **Medication-induced Postural Tremor**
333.90 **Medication-induced Movement Disorder NOS**

995.2 **Adverse Effects of Medication NOS**

Relational Problems
V61.9 **Relational Problem Related to A Mental Disorder or General Medical Condition**
V61.20 **Parent-Child Relational Problem**
V61.12 **Partner Relational Problem**
V61.8 **Sibling Relational Problem**
V62.81 **Relational Problem NOS**

Problems Related to Abuse or Neglect
V61.21 **Physical Abuse of Child**
V61.22 **Sexual Abuse of Child**
V61.21 **Neglect of Child**
V61.10 **Physical Abuse of Adult**
V51.11 **Sexual Abuse of Adult**

Additional Conditions That May Be a Focus of Clinical Attention
V62.82 **Bereavement**
V40.0 **Borderline Intellectual Functioning**
V62.3 **Academic Problem**
V62.2 **Occupational Problem**
V71.02 **Childhood or Adolescent Antisocial Behavior**
V71.01 **Adult Antisocial Behavior**
V65.2 **Malingering**
V62.89 **Phase of Life Problem**
V15.81 **Noncompliance with treatment for a mental disorder**
313.82 **Identity Problem**

V62.61	Religious or Spiritual Problem
V62.4	Acculturation Problem
780.9	Age-Associated Memory Decline

ADDITIONAL CODES

300.9	Unspecified Mental Disorder
V71.09	No Diagnosis or Condition on Axis I
799.9	Diagnosis or Condition Deferred on Axis I
V71.09	No Diagnosis on Axis II
799.9	Diagnosis Deferred on Axis II

Multiaxial Assessment

A multiaxial system involves an assessment on several axes, each of which refers to a different domain of information that may help the clinician plan treatment and predict outcome. There are five axes included in the DSM-IV multiaxial classification:

Diagnostic Axes
Axis I: Clinical Syndromes
            Other Conditions That May Be a Focus of Clinical Attention
Axis II: Personality Disorders
Axis III: General Medical Conditions

Other Domains for Assessment
Axis IV: Psychosocial and Environmental Problems
Axis V: Global Assessment of Functioning

The use of the multiaxial system facilitates comprehensive and systematic evaluation with attention to the various mental disorders and general medical conditions, social and environmental problems, and level of functioning that might be overlooked if the focus were on assessing a single presenting problem. A multiaxial system provides a convenient format for organizing and communicating clinical information, for capturing the complexity of clinical situations, and for describing the heterogeneity of individuals presenting with the same diagnosis. In addition, the multiaxial system promotes the application of the biopsychosocial model in clinical, educational, and research settings.

The rest of this section will provide a description of each of the DSM-IV axes. In some settings or situations, clinicians may prefer not to use the multiaxial system. For this reason, guidelines for reporting the results of a DSM-IV assessment without applying the formal multiaxial system are provided at the end of this section.

Axis I: Clinical Syndromes and Other Conditions That May Be a Focus of Clinical Attention

Axis I is for reporting all the various disorders in the classification except for the Personality Disorders (which are reported on Axis II). The major groups of disorders to be reported on Axis I are listed in the box below. Also reported on Axis I are Other Conditions That May be a Focus of Clinical Attention.

When an individual has more than one Axis I disorder, all of these should be reported (for examples, see page xx.) If more than one Axis I disorder is present, the principal diagnosis (see p.xx) is indicated by listing it first. When an individual has both an Axis I and an Axis II disorder, the principal diagnosis will be assumed to be on Axis I unless the Axis II diagnosis is followed by the qualifying phrase "(Principal diagnosis)." If no Axis I disorder is present, this is coded as V71.09. If an Axis I diagnosis is deferred, pending the gathering of additional information, this should be coded as 799.9.

Axis I: Clinical Syndromes and Other Conditions That May Be a Focus of Clinical Attention

Disorders Usually First Diagnosed During Infancy, Childhood or
  Adolescence
Delirium, Dementia, Amnestic and Other Cognitive Disorders
Mental Disorders Due to a General Medical Condition
Substance-Related Disorders
Schizophrenia and Other Psychotic Disorders
Mood Disorders
Anxiety Disorders
Somatoform Disorders
Factitious Disorders
Dissociative Disorders
Sexual and Gender Identity Disorders
Eating Disorders
Sleep Disorders
Impulse Control Disorders Not Elsewhere Classified
Adjustment Disorders
Other Conditions That May Be a Focus of Clinical Attention

Axis II: Personality Disorders

Axis II is for reporting Personality Disorders, and may also be used for noting prominent maladaptive personality features, and defense mechanisms. The provision of a separate axis for Personality Disorders ensures that consideration be given to the possible presence of Personality Disorders that might otherwise be overlooked when attention is directed to the usually more florid Axis I disorders. The coding of Personality Disorders on Axis II should not be taken to imply that their pathogenesis or range of appropriate treatment is fundamentally different from the disorders coded on Axis I. The Personality Disorders to be reported on Axis II are listed in the box below.

In the common situation in which an individual has more than one Axis II diagnosis, all should be reported (for examples, see page xx.) When an individual has both an Axis I and an Axis II diagnosis and the Axis II diagnosis is the principal diagnosis, this is indicated by adding the qualifying phrase "(Principal diagnosis)" after the Axis II diagnosis. If no Axis II disorder is present, this is coded as V71.09. If an Axis II diagnosis is deferred, pending the gathering of additional information, this should be coded as 799.9.

Axis II may also be used to indicate specific maladaptive personality features that do not meet the threshold for a Personality Disorder (in such instances, no code number should be used--see example 3 on page D:9). The habitual use of particular defense mechanisms may also be indicated on Axis II (see Glossary p.xx for definitions and example 1 on page D:9).

Axis II: Personality Disorders

Paranoid Personality Disorder
Schizoid Personality Disorder
Schizotypal Personality Disorder
Antisocial Personality Disorder
Borderline Personality Disorder
Histrionic Personality Disorder
Narcissistic Personality Disorder
Avoidant Personality Disorder
Dependent Personality Disorder
Obsessive-Compulsive Personality Disorder
Personality Disorder Not Otherwise Specified

Axis III: General Medical Conditions

Axis III is for reporting current general medical conditions that are potentially relevant to the understanding or management of the case. These conditions are classified outside the mental disorders section of ICD-9-CM (and outside Chapter F of ICD-10). A listing of the broad categories of general medical conditions is given in the box below. (For a more detailed listing, refer to Appendix G.)

As discussed in the Use of the Manual, the multiaxial distinction among Axis I, II, and III disorders does not imply that there are fundamental differences in their conceptualization, or that mental disorders are unrelated to physical or biological factors or processes, or that general medical conditions are unrelated to behavioral or psychosocial factors or processes. The purpose of distinguishing general medical conditions is to encourage thoroughness in evaluation and to enhance communication among health care providers.

General medical conditions can be related to mental disorders in a variety of ways. In some cases it is clear that the general medical condition is etiologic to the development or worsening of a mental disorder and that the mechanism for this effect is physiologic. When a general medical condition is judged to be etiologically related to the mental disorder, a Mental Disorder Due to a General Medical Condition is listed on Axis I and the general medical condition is listed both on Axis I and Axis III. For example, when hypothyroidism is a direct cause of Major Depressive Disorder, the designation on Axis I is 293.83 Mood Disorder due to hypothyroidism with depressive features, and the hypothyroidism is listed again and coded on Axis III as 244.9. For a further discussion, see page xx.

In those instances in which the etiologic relationship between the general medical condition and the mental disorder is insufficiently clear to warrant an Axis I diagnosis of Mental Disorder Due to a General Medical Condition, only the pertinent mental disorder (e.g., Major Depressive Disorder) is coded on Axis I; the general medical condition is listed and coded on Axis III.

There are other situations in which general medical conditions should be recorded on Axis III because they are important in the overall understanding or treatment of the individual with the mental disorder. An Axis I disorder may be a psychological reaction to an Axis III general medical condition (e.g., the development of 309.00 Adjustment Disorder with Depressed Mood as a reaction to the diagnosis of carcinoma of the breast). Some general medical conditions may not be directly related to the mental disorder but nonetheless have important prognostic or treatment implications (e.g., a case with both 296.2 Major Depressive Disorder on Axis I and 427.9 arrhythmia on Axis III, in which the choice of pharmacotherapy is influenced by the general medical condition; a person with diabetes mellitus admitted to the hospital for an exacerbation of Schizophrenia for whom insulin management must be monitored).

When an individual has more than one Axis III diagnosis, all should be reported. For examples, see page xx. If no Axis III disorder is present, this should be indicated by "Axis III: None." If an Axis III diagnosis is deferred, pending the gathering of additional information, this should be indicated by "Axis III: Deferred."

Axis III: ICD-9-CM General Medical Conditions

Infectious and Parasitic Diseases (001-139)
Neoplasms (140-239)
Endocrine, Nutritional, and Metabolic Diseases and Immunity Disorders
  (240-279)
Diseases of the Blood and Blood-Forming Organs (280-289)
Diseases of the Nervous and Sense Organs (320-389)
Diseases of the Circulatory System (390-459)
Diseases of the Respiratory System (460-519)
Diseases of the Digestive System (520-579)
Diseases of the Genitourinary System (580-629)
Complications of Pregnancy, Childbirth, and the Puerperium (630-676)
Diseases of the Skin and Subcutaneous Tissue (680-709)
Diseases of the Musculoskeletal System and Connective Tissue (710-739)
Congenital Anomalies (740-759)
Certain Conditions Originating in the Perinatal Period (760-779)
Symptoms, Signs, and Ill-Defined Conditions (780-799)
Injury and Poisoning (800-999)

Axis IV: Psychosocial and Environmental Problems

Axis IV is for reporting psychosocial and environmental problems that may affect the diagnosis, treatment, and prognosis of mental disorders (Axis I and II). A psychosocial or environmental problem may be a negative life event, an environmental difficulty or deficiency, a familial or other interpersonal stress, an inadequacy of social support or personal resources, or another problem that describes the context in which a person's difficulties have developed. So-called positive stressors, such as job promotion, should be listed only if they constitute or create a problem, as when a person has difficulty adapting to the new situation. In addition to playing a role in the initiation or exacerbation of a mental disorder, psychosocial problems may also develop as a consequence of a person's psychopathology, or may constitute problems that should be considered in the overall management plan.

The following problem categories may be noted on Axis IV; each is followed by a list of examples:

Problems with Primary Support Group (Childhood [V61.9], Adult [V61.9], Parent-Child [V61.2]). These include: death of a family member; health problems in family; disruption of family by separation, divorce, or estrangement; removal from the home; remarriage of parent; sexual or physical abuse; parental overprotection; neglect of child; inadequate discipline; discord with siblings; birth of a sibling.

Problems Related to the Social Environment (V62.4). These include: death or loss of friend; social isolation; living alone; difficulty with acculturation; discrimination; adjustment to life cycle transition (e.g., retirement).

Educational Problems (V62.3). These include: illiteracy; academic problems; discord with teachers or classmates; inadequate school environment.

Occupational Problems (V62.2). These include: unemployment; threat of job loss; stressful work schedule; difficult work condition; job dissatisfaction; job change; discord with boss or coworkers.

Housing Problems (V60.9). These include: homelessness; inadequate housing; unsafe neighborhood; discord with neighbors or landlord.

Economic Problems (V60.9). These include: extreme poverty; inadequate finances; insufficient welfare support.

Problems with Access to Health Care Services (V63.9). These include: inadequate health care services; transportation to health care facilities unavailable; inadequate health insurance.

Problems Related to Interaction with the Legal System/Crime (V62.5). These include: arrest; incarceration; litigation; victim of crime.

Other Psychosocial Problems (V62.9). These include: exposure to disasters, war, other hostilities; discord with non-family caregivers (e.g., counselor, social worker, physician); unavailability of social service agencies.

When using the multiaxial recording form (see box below and page xx), the clinician should identify the relevant categories of psychosocial or environmental problems and indicate the specific factors involved. If a recording form with a checklist of problems is not used, the clinician may simply list the specific problems on Axis IV. (See examples p.xx.)

When an individual has multiple psychosocial or environmental problems, the clinician may note as many as are judged to be relevant. In general, the clinician should note only those psychosocial and environmental problems that have been present during the year preceding the current evaluation. However, the clinician may choose to note psychosocial and environmental problems occurring prior to the previous year if these are clearly contributory to the mental disorder or have become a focus of treatment, e.g., previous combat experiences leading to Posttraumatic Stress Disorder.

In practice, most psychosocial and environmental problems will be indicated on Axis IV. However, when a psychosocial or environmental problem is the primary focus of clinical attention, it should also be recorded on Axis I with a code derived from the section on Other Conditions That May Be a Focus of Clinical Attention (see p. xx).

Axis IV: Psychosocial and Environmental Problems

Check:
___ Problems with primary support group (Childhood [V61.9], Adult [V61.9], Parent-Child [V61.2]). Specify: _____
___ Problems related to the social environment (V62.4). Specify: _____
___ Educational problem (V62.3). Specify: _____
___ Occupational problem (V62.2). Specify: _____
___ Housing problem (V60.9). Specify: _____
___ Economic problem (V60.9). Specify: _____
___ Problems with access to health care services (V63.9). Specify: _____
___ Problems related to interaction with the legal system/crime (V62.5). Specify: _____
___ Other psychosocial problem (V62.9). Specify: _____

Axis V: Global Assessment of Functioning

Axis V is for reporting the clinician's judgment of the individual's overall level of functioning. This information is useful in planning treatment and measuring its impact, and in predicting outcome.

The reporting of overall functioning on Axis V can be done using the **Global Assessment of Functioning (GAF) Scale**. The GAF Scale may be particularly useful in tracking the clinical progress of individuals in global terms, using a single measure. A suggested method for recording the scores in a multiaxial format is given on p.xx. The GAF Scale is to be rated with respect only to psychological, social, and occupational functioning. The instructions specify, "Do not include impairment in functioning due to physical (or environmental) limitations." In most instances, the GAF Scale should be rated for the current period (i.e., the level of functioning at the time of the evaluation) because ratings of current functioning will generally reflect the need for treatment or care. In some settings, the GAF Scale may also be rated for other time periods (i.e., the highest level of functioning for at least a few months during the past year).

In some settings, it may be useful to assess social and occupational disability and track progress in rehabilitation independent of the severity of the psychological symptoms. For this purpose, a proposed Social and Occupational Functioning Assessment Scale (SOFAS) is included in the Appendix (see page xx). Two additional proposed scales (Global Assessment of Relational Functioning [GARF] and Defensive Styles Rating Scale) that may be useful in some settings are included in the Appendix (see page xx).

Global Assessment of Functioning (GAF) Scale[1]

Consider psychological, social, and occupational functioning on a hypothetical continuum of mental health-illness. Do not include impairment in functioning due to physical (or environmental) limitations.

Code (Note: Use intermediate codes when appropriate, e.g., 45, 68, 72.)

100 | **Superior functioning in a wide range of activities, life's problems never seem to get out of hand, is sought out by others because of his many positive qualities. No symptoms.**
91

90 | **Absent or minimal symptoms** (e.g., mild anxiety before an exam), **good functioning in all areas, interested and involved in a wide range of activities, socially effective, generally satisfied with life, no more than everyday problems or concerns** (e.g., an occasional argument with
81 | family members).

80 | **If symptoms are present, they are transient and expectable reactions to psychosocial stressors** (e.g., difficulty concentrating after family argument); **no more than slight impairment in social, occupational, or**
71 | **school functioning** (e.g., temporarily falling behind in school work).

70 | **Some mild symptoms** (e.g., depressed mood and mild insomnia) **OR some difficulty in social, occupational, or school functioning** (e.g., occasional truancy, or theft within the household), **but generally functioning**
61 | **pretty well, has some meaningful interpersonal relationships.**

60 | **Moderate symptoms** (e.g., flat affect and circumstantial speech, occasional panic attacks) **OR moderate difficulty in social, occupational, or school**
51 | **functioning** (e.g., no friends, unable to keep a job).

50 | **Serious symptoms** (e.g., suicidal ideation, severe obsessional rituals, frequent shoplifting) **OR any serious impairment in social, occupational,**
41 | **or school functioning** (e.g., no friends, unable to keep a job).

40 | **Some impairment in reality testing or communication** (e.g., speech is at times illogical, obscure, or irrelevant) **OR major impairment in several areas, such as work or school, family relations, judgment, thinking, or mood** (e.g., depressed man avoids friends, neglects family, and is unable to work; child frequently
31 | beats up younger children, is defiant at home, and is failing at school).

30 | **Behavior is considerably influenced by delusions or hallucinations OR serious impairment in communication or judgment** (e.g.,sometimes incoherent, acts grossly inappropriately, suicidal preoccupation) **OR inability to function**
21 | **in almost all areas** (e.g., stays in bed all day; no job, home, or friends).

20 | **Some danger of hurting self or others** (e.g., suicide attempts without clear expectation of death, frequently violent, manic excitement) **OR occasionally fails to maintain minimal personal hygiene** (e.g., smears feces) **OR gross**
11 | **impairment in communication** (e.g., largely incoherent or mute).

10 | **Persistent danger of severely hurting self or others** (e.g., recurrent violence) **OR persistent inability to maintain minimal personal hygiene OR**
1 | **serious suicidal act with clear expectation of death.**

0 | **Inadequate information.**

[1] The GAF Scale is a revision of the GAS (Endicott J, Spitzer RL, Fleiss, et al: The Global Assessment Scale: A procedure for measuring overall severity of psychiatric disturbance. Archives of General Psychiatry 33:766-771, 1976) and the CGAS (Shaffer D, Gould MS, Brasic J, et al: Children's Global Assessment Scale (CGAS). Archives of General Psychiatry 40:1228-1231, 1983). These are revisions of the Global Scale of the Health-Sickness Rating Scale (Luborsky L: Clinicians' judgments of mental health. Archives of General Psychiatry 7:407-417, 1962).

Examples of How To Record the Results of a DSM-IV Multiaxial Evaluation

Example 1:

Axis I:	296.23	Major Depressive Disorder, single episode, severe but without psychotic features
	305.0	Alcohol abuse
Axis II:	301.6	Dependent Personality Disorder
		Frequent use of denial
Axis III:	None	
Axis IV:	V62.2	Occupational problem (threat of job loss)
Axis V:	GAF = 35	

Example 2:

Axis I:	300.4	Dysthymic Disorder
	315.0	Reading disorder
Axis II:	V71.09	No diagnosis on Axis II
Axis III:	382.9	Otitis media, recurrent
Axis IV:	V61.2	Parent-child problem (neglect of child)
Axis V:	GAF = 53	

Example 3:

Axis I:	293.83	Mood Disorder due to hypothyroidism, with depressive features
Axis II:	V71.09	No diagnosis on Axis II, histrionic personality features
Axis III:	244.9	Hypothyroidism
	365.11	Chronic-angle closure glaucoma
Axis IV:	None	
Axis V:	GAF = 45	

Example 4:

Axis I:	V61.12	Partner Relational Problem
Axis II:	V71.09	No diagnosis on Axis II
Axis III:	None	
Axis IV:	V62.2	Occupational Problem (unemployment)
Axis V:	GAF = 83	

Multiaxial Evaluation Report Form

The following is offered as one possible form for reporting multiaxial evaluations. In some settings, this form may be used exactly as is; in other settings, the form may be adapted to satisfy special needs.

AXIS I: CLINICAL SYNDROMES
OTHER CONDITIONS THAT MAY BE A FOCUS OF CLINICAL ATTENTION

DSM-IV Code   DSM-IV Name

_ _ _._ _   _____

_ _ _._ _   _____

_ _ _._ _   _____

AXIS II: PERSONALITY DISORDERS

DSM-IV Code   DSM-IV Name

_ _ _._ _   _____

_ _ _._ _   _____

AXIS III: GENERAL MEDICAL CONDITIONS

ICD-9-CM Code   ICD-9-CM Name

_ _ _._ _   _____

_ _ _._ _   _____

_ _ _._ _   _____

AXIS IV: PSYCHOSOCIAL AND ENVIRONMENTAL PROBLEMS

Check:
___ Problems with primary support group (Childhood [V61.9], Adult [V61.9], Parent-Child [V61.2]). Specify: _____
___ Problems related to the social environment (V62.4). Specify: _____
___ Educational problem (V62.3). Specify: _____
___ Occupational problem (V62.2). Specify: _____
___ Housing problem (V60.9). Specify: _____
___ Economic problem (V60.9). Specify: _____
___ Problems with access to health care services (V63.9). Specify: _____
___ Problems related to interaction with the legal system/crime (V62.5). Specify: _____
___ Other psychosocial problem (V62.9). Specify: _____

AXIS V: GLOBAL ASSESSMENT OF FUNCTIONING SCALE   Code: _ _

Nonaxial Format

Clinicians who do not wish to use the multiaxial format may simply list the appropriate diagnoses.   Those choosing this option should follow the general rule of recording as many co-existing mental disorders, general medical conditions, and other factors that are relevant to the care and treatment of the individual. The principal diagnosis should be listed first.

The examples below illustrate the reporting of diagnoses in a format that does not use the multiaxial system.

Example 1:
296.23   Major depressive disorder, single episode, severe but without psychotic features
305.0   Alcohol abuse
301.6   Dependent Personality Disorder
          Frequent use of denial

Example 2:
300.4   Dysthymic Disorder
315.0   Reading disorder
382.9   Otitis media, recurrent

Example 3:
293.83   Mood disorder due to hypothyroidism, with depressive features
244.9   Hypothyroidism
365.11   Chronic-angle closure glaucoma
          Histrionic personality features

Example 4:
V61.12   Partner relational problem

Disorders Usually First Diagnosed in Infancy, Childhood, or Adolescence

Mental Retardation

A. Significantly subaverage intellectual functioning: an IQ of approximately 70 or below on an individually administered IQ test (for infants, a clinical judgment of significantly subaverage intellectual functioning).

B. Concurrent deficits or impairments in present adaptive functioning (i.e., the person's effectiveness in meeting the standards expected for his or her age by his or her cultural group, in at least two of the following skill areas: communication, self-care, home living, social/interpersonal skills, use of community resources, self-direction, functional academic skills, work, leisure, health and safety).

C. Onset before the age of 18.

Code based on degree of severity reflecting level of intellectual impairment:

317   **Mild Mental Retardation**: IQ level 50-55 to approximately 70
318.0   **Moderate Retardation**: IQ level 35-40 to 50-55
318.1   **Severe Mental Retardation**: IQ level 20-25 to 35-40
318.2   **Profound Mental Retardation**: IQ level below 20 or 25
319   **Mental Retardation, Severity Unspecified:** when there is a strong presumption of Mental Retardation but the person is untestable by standard intelligence tests.

Learning Disorders (Academic Skills Disorders)

315.00 Reading Disorder (Developmental Reading Disorder)

A. Reading achievement, as measured by an individually administered standardized test of reading accuracy or comprehension, is substantially below that expected given the person's chronological age, measured intelligence, and age-appropriate education.

B. The disturbance in A significantly interferes with academic achievement or activities of daily living that require reading skills.

C. If a sensory deficit is present, the learning difficulties are in excess of those usually associated with it.

Coding note: if a general medical (e.g., neurological) condition or sensory deficit is present, code the condition on Axis III.

E:1

315.1 Mathematics Disorder (Developmental Arithmetic Disorder)

A.   Mathematical ability, as measured by an individually administered standardized test, is substantially below that expected given the person's chronological age, measured intelligence, and age-appropriate education.

B.   The disturbance in A significantly interferes with academic achievement or activities of daily living that require mathematical ability.

C.   If a sensory deficit is present, the learning difficulties are in excess of those usually associated with it.

Coding note: if a general medical (e.g., neurological) condition or sensory deficit is present, code the condition on Axis III.

315.2 Disorder of Written Expression (Developmental Expressive Writing Disorder)

A.   Writing skills, as measured by an individually administered standardized test (or functional assessment of writing skills), are substantially below that expected given the person's chronological age, measured intelligence, and age-appropriate education.

B.   The disturbance in A significantly interferes with academic achievement or activities of daily living that require the composition of written texts (e.g., writing grammatically correct sentences and organized paragraphs).

C.   If a sensory deficit is present, the learning difficulties are in excess of those usually associated it.

Coding note: if a general medical (e.g., neurological) condition or sensory deficit is present, code the condition on Axis III.

315.9 Learning Disorder Not Otherwise Specified

This category is for disorders in learning that do not meet criteria for any specific Learning Disorder. For example, a disorder in which spelling skills are substantially below that expected given the person's chronological age, measured intelligence, and age-appropriate education.

Motor Skills Disorder

315.4 Developmental Coordination Disorder

A. Performance in daily activities that require motor coordination is substantially below that expected given the person's chronological age and measured intelligence. This may be manifested by marked delays in achieving motor milestones (e.g., walking, crawling, sitting), dropping things, "clumsiness," poor performance in sports, or poor handwriting.

B. The disturbance in A significantly interferes with academic achievement or activities of daily living.

C. Not due to a general medical condition (e.g., cerebral palsy, hemiplegia, or muscular dystrophy).

Pervasive Developmental Disorders

299.0 Autistic Disorder

A. A total of at least six items from (1), (2), and (3), with at least two from (1), and one each from (2) and (3):

(1) Qualitative impairment in social interaction, as manifested by at least two of the following:

(a) marked impairment in the use of multiple nonverbal behaviors such as eye-to-eye gaze, facial expression, body postures, and gestures to regulate social interaction

(b) failure to develop peer relationships appropriate to developmental level

(c) markedly impaired expression of pleasure in other people's happiness

(d) lack of social or emotional reciprocity

(2) Qualitative impairments in communication as manifested by at least one of the following:

    (a) delay in, or total lack of, the development of spoken language (not accompanied by an attempt to compensate through alternative modes of communication such as gesture or mime)

    (b) in individuals with adequate speech, marked impairment in the ability to initiate or sustain a conversation with others

    (c) stereotyped and repetitive use of language or idiosyncratic language

    (d) lack of varied spontaneous make-believe play or social imitative play appropriate to developmental level

(3) Restricted repetitive and stereotyped patterns of behavior, interests, and activities, as manifested by at least one of the following:

    (a) encompassing preoccupation with one or more stereotyped and restricted patterns of interest that is abnormal either in intensity or focus

    (b) apparently compulsive adherence to specific, nonfunctional routines or rituals

    (c) stereotyped and repetitive motor mannerisms (e.g., hand or finger flapping or twisting, or complex whole body movements)

    (d) persistent preoccupation with parts of objects

B. Delays or abnormal functioning in at least one of the following areas, with onset prior to age three: (1) social interaction, (2) language as used in social communication, or (3) symbolic or imaginative play.

C. Not better accounted for by Rett's Disorder or Childhood Disintegrative Disorder.

299.80 Rett's Disorder

A. Normal development for at least the first six months as manifested by all of the following:

(1) apparently normal prenatal and perinatal development

(2) apparently normal psychomotor development through the first six months

(3) normal head circumference at birth

B.   Onset of all of the following between 5 and 48 months:

(1)   deceleration of head growth

(2)   loss of previously acquired purposeful hand movements, with the development of stereotyped hand movements (e.g., handwringing or handwashing)

(3)   loss of social engagement early in the course (although often social interaction develops later)

(4)   appearance of poorly coordinated gait or trunk movements

(5)   marked delay and impairment of expressive and receptive language with severe psychomotor retardation

299.10 Childhood Disintegrative Disorder

A.   Apparently normal development for at least the first two years as manifested by the presence of age-appropriate verbal and non-verbal communication, social relationships, play, and adaptive behavior.

B.   Clinically significant loss of previously acquired skills in at least two of the following areas:

(1)   expressive or receptive language

(2)   social skills or adaptive behavior

(3)   bowel or bladder control

(4)   play

(5)   motor skills

C. Abnormalities of functioning in at least two of the following areas:

    (1) Qualitative impairment in social interaction, as manifested by at least two of the following:

        (a) marked impairment in the use of multiple nonverbal behaviors such as eye-to-eye gaze, facial expression, body postures, and gestures to regulate social interaction

        (b) failure to develop peer relationships appropriate to developmental level

        (c) markedly impaired expression of pleasure in other people's happiness

        (d) lack of social or emotional reciprocity

    (2) Qualitative impairments in communication as manifested by at least one of the following:

        (a) delay in, or total lack of, the development of spoken language (not accompanied by an attempt to compensate through alternative modes of communication such as gesture or mime)

        (b) in individuals with adequate speech, marked impairment in the ability to initiate or sustain a conversation with others

        (c) stereotyped and repetitive use of language or idiosyncratic language

        (d) lack of varied spontaneous make-believe play or social imitative play appropriate to developmental level

    (3) restricted, repetitive, and stereotyped patterns of behavior, interests, and activities, including motor stereotypies and mannerisms

D. Not better accounted for by another specific Pervasive Developmental Disorder or by Schizophrenia.

Asperger's Disorder (placement in classification vs. Appendix has not been decided)

A.   Qualitative impairment in social interaction, as manifested by at least two of the following:

(1)   marked impairment in the use of multiple nonverbal behaviors such as eye-to-eye gaze, facial expression, body postures, and gestures to regulate social interaction

(2)   failure to develop peer relationships appropriate to developmental level

(3)   markedly impaired expression of pleasure in other people's happiness

(4)   lack of social or emotional reciprocity

B.   Restricted, repetitive, and stereotyped patterns of behavior, interests, and activities.

C.   Lack of any clinically significant general delay in language (e.g., single words used by age two, communicative phrases used by age three).

D.   Lack of any clinically significant delay in cognitive development as manifested by the development of age-appropriate self-help skills, adaptive behavior, and curiosity about the environment.

E.   Does not meet criteria for another specific Pervasive Developmental Disorder.

299.80 Pervasive Developmental Disorder Not Otherwise Specified (including Atypical Autism)

This category should be used when there is a severe and pervasive impairment in the development of reciprocal social interaction, verbal and nonverbal communication skills, or the development of stereotyped behavior, interests, and activities, but the criteria are not met for a specific Pervasive Developmental Disorder, Schizophrenia, Schizotypal Personality Disorder, or Avoidant Personality Disorder. Examples include:

1)   Atypical autism: cases that do not meet the criteria for Autistic Disorder because of late age at onset, atypical symptomatology, or subthreshold symptomatology, or all of these.

2)   Asperger's disorder: gross and sustained impairment in social interaction and restricted, repetitive, and stereotyped patterns of behavior, interests, and activities, occurring in the context of preserved cognitive and language development. (See page xx for suggested criteria).

Disruptive Behavior and Attention-deficit Disorders

Attention-deficit/Hyperactivity Disorder

A. Either (1) or (2):

    (1) Inattention: At least six of the following symptoms of inattention have persisted for at least six months to a degree that is maladaptive and inconsistent with developmental level:

        (a) often fails to give close attention to details or makes careless mistakes in schoolwork, work, or other activities

        (b) often has difficulty sustaining attention in tasks or play activities

        (c) often does not seem to listen to what is being said to him or her

        (d) often does not follow through on instructions and fails to finish schoolwork, chores, or duties in the workplace (not due to oppositional behavior or failure to understand instructions)

        (e) often has difficulties organizing tasks and activities

        (f) often avoids or strongly dislikes tasks (such as schoolwork or homework) that require sustained mental effort

        (g) often loses things necessary for tasks or activities (e.g., school assignments, pencils, books, tools, or toys)

        (h) is often easily distracted by extraneous stimuli

        (i) often forgetful in daily activities

    (2) Hyperactivity-Impulsivity: At least four of the following symptoms of hyperactivity-impulsivity have persisted for at least six months to a degree that is maladaptive and inconsistent with developmental level:

    Hyperactivity

        (a) often fidgets with hands or feet or squirms in seat

        (b) leaves seat in classroom or in other situations in which remaining seated is expected

        (c) often runs about or climbs excessively in situations where it is inappropriate (in adolescents or adults, may be limited to subjective feelings of restlessness)

        (d)   often has difficulty playing or engaging in leisure activities quietly

      <u>Impulsivity</u>

        (e)   often blurts out answers to questions before the questions have been completed

        (f)   often has difficulty waiting in lines or awaiting turn in games or group situations

B.   Onset no later than seven years of age.

C.   Symptoms must be present in two or more situations (e.g., at school, work, and at home).

D.   The disturbance causes clinically significant distress or impairment in social, academic, or occupational functioning.

E.   Does not occur exclusively during the course of a Pervasive Developmental Disorder, Schizophrenia or other Psychotic Disorder, and is not better accounted for by a Mood Disorder, Anxiety Disorder, Dissociative Disorder, or a Personality Disorder.

Code based on type:

314.00 Attention-deficit/Hyperactivity Disorder, Predominantly Inattentive Type: if criterion A(1) is met but not criterion A(2) for the past six months

314.01 Attention-deficit/Hyperactivity Disorder, Predominantly Hyperactive-Impulsive Type: if criterion A(2) is met but not criterion A(1) for the past six months

314.01 Attention-deficit/Hyperactivity Disorder, Combined Type: if both criteria A(1) and A(2) are met for the past six months

Coding note: for individuals (especially adolescents and adults) who currently have symptoms that no longer meet full criteria, "in partial remission" should be specified.

314.9 Attention-deficit/Hyperactivity Disorder Not Otherwise Specified

This category is for disorders with prominent symptoms of attention-deficit or hyperactivity-impulsivity that do not meet criteria for Attention Deficit/Hyperactivity Disorder.

312.8 Conduct Disorder

A. A repetitive and persistent pattern of behavior in which either the basic rights of others or major age-appropriate societal norms or rules are violated, lasting at least six months, during which at least three of the following are present:

(1) often bullies, threatens, or intimidates others

(2) often initiates physical fights

(3) has used a weapon that can cause serious physical harm to others (e.g., a bat, brick, broken bottle, knife, gun)

(4) has stolen with confrontation with a victim (e.g., mugging, purse snatching, extortion, armed robbery)

(5) has been physically cruel to people

(6) has been physically cruel to animals

(7) has forced someone into sexual activity

(8) often lies or breaks promises to obtain goods or favors or to avoid obligations (i.e., "cons" others)

(9) often stays out at night despite parental prohibitions, beginning before 13 years of age

(10) has stolen items of nontrivial value without confrontation with the victim either within the home or outside the home (e.g., shoplifting, burglary, forgery)

(11) has deliberately engaged in fire setting with the intention of causing serious damage

(12) has deliberately destroyed others' property (other than by fire setting)

(13) has run away from home overnight at least twice while living in parental or parental surrogate home (or once without returning for a lengthy period)

(14) often truant from school, beginning before 13 years of age (for employed person, absent from work)

(15) has broken into someone else's house, building, or car

B. If age 18 or older, does not meet criteria for Antisocial Personality Disorder.

Specify type based on age of onset:

Childhood onset type: onset of at least one conduct problem prior to age 10.
Adolescent onset type: no conduct problems prior to age 10.

Specify severity:

Mild: Few if any conduct problems in excess of those required to make the diagnosis, **and** conduct problems cause only minor harm to others.

Moderate: Number of conduct problems and effect on others intermediate between "mild" and "severe"

Severe: Many conduct problems in excess of those required to make the diagnosis, **or** conduct problems cause considerable harm to others, e.g., serious physical injury to victims, extensive vandalism or theft.

313.81 Oppositional Defiant Disorder

A.   A pattern of negativistic, hostile, and defiant behavior lasting at least six months, during which at least four of the following are present:

    (1)   often loses temper

    (2)   often argues with adults

    (3)   often actively defies or refuses to comply with adults' requests or rules

    (4)   often deliberately does things that annoy other people

    (5)   often blames others for his or her mistakes or misbehavior

    (6)   is often touchy or easily annoyed by others

    (7)   is often angry and resentful

    (8)   is often spiteful or vindictive

B.   The disturbance in behavior causes significant impairment in social, academic or occupational functioning.

C.   Does not occur exclusively during the course of a Psychotic or Mood Disorder.

D.   Does not meet criteria for Conduct Disorder and, if 18 or older, does not meet criteria for Antisocial Personality Disorder.

312.9 Disruptive Behavior Disorder Not Otherwise Specified

This category is for disorders characterized by conduct or oppositional-defiant behaviors that do not meet the criteria for Conduct Disorder or Oppositional Defiant Disorder. For example, include clinical presentations that are subthreshold for both Oppositional Defiant Disorder and Conduct Disorder, but in which there is clinically significant impairment.

Feeding and Eating Disorders of Infancy or Early Childhood

307.52 Pica

A.   Persistent eating of nonnutritive substances for at least one month.

B.   The eating of nonnutritive substances is inappropriate to developmental level.

C.   The eating behavior is not part of a culturally sanctioned practice.

307.53 Rumination Disorder

A.   Repeated regurgitation and rechewing of food (in the absence of associated gastrointestinal illness) for a period of at least one month following a period of normal functioning.

B.   Not due to an associated gastrointestinal or other general medical condition (e.g., esophageal reflux).

307.59 Feeding Disorder of Infancy or Early Childhood

A.   Feeding disturbance as manifested by persistent failure to eat adequately with significant failure to gain weight or significant loss of weight over at least one month.

B.   Not due to an associated gastrointestinal or other general medical condition (e.g., esophageal reflux).

C.   Not better accounted for by another mental disorder or by lack of available food.

D.   Onset before age six.

Tic Disorders

307.23 Tourette's Disorder

A. Both multiple motor and one or more vocal tics have been present at some time during the illness, although not necessarily concurrently. (A tic is an involuntary, sudden, rapid, recurrent, nonrhythmic, stereotyped motor movement or vocalization.)

B. The tics occur many times a day (usually in bouts), nearly every day or intermittently throughout a period of more than one year; (?) and during this period, never without tics for more than two months at a time.

C. Onset before age 18.

D. Not due to the direct effects of a substance (e.g., stimulants) or a general medical condition (e.g., Huntington's chorea or postviral encephalitis).

307.22 Chronic Motor or Vocal Tic Disorder

A. Either vocal or motor tics (i.e., involuntary, sudden, rapid, recurrent, nonrhythmic, stereotyped motor movements or vocalizations) but not both, have been present at some time during the illness.

B. The tics occur many times a day, nearly every day or intermittently throughout a period of more than one year; (?) and during this period, never without tics for more than two months at a time.

C. Onset before age 18.

D. Has never met the criteria for Tourette's Disorder.

E. Not due to a substance (e.g., stimulants) or a general medical condition (e.g., Huntington's chorea or postviral encephalitis).

307.21 Transient Tic Disorder

A. Single or multiple motor or vocal tics (i.e., involuntary, sudden, rapid, recurrent, nonrhythmic, stereotyped motor movements or vocalizations)

B. The tics occur many times a day, nearly every day for at least four weeks, for no longer than 12 consecutive months.

C. Onset before age 18.

D. Has never met the criteria for Tourette's or Chronic Motor or Vocal Tic Disorder.

E.   Not due to a substance (e.g., stimulants) or a general medical condition (e.g., Huntington's chorea or postviral encephalitis).

Specify if: **Single Episode** or **Recurrent**

307.20 Tic Disorder Not Otherwise Specified

This category is for a tic disorder that does not meet criteria for a specific Tic Disorder.

Communication Disorders

315.31 Expressive Language Disorder (Developmental Expressive Language Disorder)

A.   The scores obtained from standardized measures of expressive language development are substantially below those obtained from standardized measures of both nonverbal intellectual capacity and receptive language development. The disturbance may be manifest clinically by having a markedly limited vocabulary, making errors in tense, or having difficulty recalling words or producing sentences with developmentally appropriate length or complexity.

B.   The difficulties with expressive language interfere with academic or occupational achievement, or with social communication.

C.   Does not does meet criteria for Mixed Receptive/Expressive Language Disorder or a Pervasive Developmental Disorder.

D.   If Mental Retardation, a speech-motor or sensory deficit, or environmental deprivation is present, the language difficulties are in excess of those usually associated with these problems.

Coding note: if a speech-motor or sensory deficit or a neurological condition is present, code the condition on Axis III.

315.31 Mixed Receptive/Expressive Language Disorder (Developmental Receptive Language Disorder)

A.   The scores obtained from a battery of standardized measures of both receptive and expressive language development are substantially below those obtained from standardized measures of nonverbal intellectual capacity. Symptoms include those for Expressive Language Disorder as well as difficulty understanding words, sentences, or specific types of words, such as spatial terms.

B.   The difficulties with receptive and expressive language interfere with academic or occupational achievement, or with social communication.

C. Does not does meet criteria for a Pervasive Developmental Disorder.

D. If Mental Retardation, a speech-motor or sensory deficit, or environmental deprivation is present, the language difficulties are in excess of those usually associated with these problems.

Coding note: if a speech-motor or sensory deficit or a neurological condition is present, code the condition on Axis III.

315.39 Phonological Disorder (Articulation Disorder)

A. Failure to use developmentally expected speech sounds that are appropriate for age or dialect (e.g., errors in sound production, use, representation or organization such as, but not limited to, substitutions of one sound for another [use of /t/ for target /k/ sound] or omissions of sounds such as final consonants).

B. The difficulties in speech sound production interfere with academic or occupational achievement, or with social communication.

C. If Mental Retardation, a speech-motor or sensory deficit, or environmental deprivation is present, the language difficulties are in excess of those usually associated with these problems.

Coding note: if a speech-motor or sensory deficit or a neurological condition is present, code the condition on Axis III.

307.0 Stuttering

A. Disturbance in the normal fluency and time patterning of speech (inappropriate for the individual's age), characterized by frequent occurrences of one or more of the following:

(1) sound and syllable repetitions

(2) sound prolongations

(3) interjections

(4) broken words (e.g., pause within a word)

(5) audible or silent blocking

(6) circumlocutions (word substitutions to avoid problematic words)

(7) words produced with an excess of physical tension

(8) monosyllabic whole word repetitions (e.g., "I-I-I-I-see him.")

B.   The disturbance in fluency interferes with academic or occupational achievement, or with social communication.

C.   If a speech-motor or sensory deficit is present, the language difficulties are in excess of those usually associated with these problems.

Coding note: if a speech-motor or sensory deficit or a neurological condition is present, code the condition on Axis III.

315.39 Communication Disorder Not Otherwise Specified

This category is for disorders in communication that do not meet criteria for any specific Communication Disorder. For example, a Voice Disorder (i.e., an abnormality of vocal pitch, loudness, quality, tone, or resonance).

Elimination Disorders

307.7 Encopresis

A.   Repeated passage of feces into inappropriate places (e.g., clothing or floor) whether involuntary or intentional.

B.   At least one such event a month for at least three months.

C.   Chronological age of at least four years (or equivalent developmental level).

D.   Not due to the direct effect of a general medical condition.

Specify type:
   with constipation and overflow incontinence
   without constipation and overflow incontinence

307.6 Enuresis

A.   Repeated voiding of urine into bed or clothes (whether involuntary or intentional).

B.   Chronological age of at least five years (or equivalent developmental level).

C.   The behavior is clinically significant as manifested by either a frequency of twice a week for at least three consecutive months, or the presence of clinically significant distress or impairment in social, academic (occupational), or other important areas of functioning.

D.   Not due to the direct effect of a general medical condition (e.g., diabetes, spina bifida, a seizure disorder).

Specify type:
   Nocturnal Only
   Diurnal Only
   Nocturnal and Diurnal

Other Disorders of Infancy, Childhood, or Adolescence

309.21 Separation Anxiety Disorder

A.   Developmentally inappropriate and excessive anxiety concerning separation from home or from those to whom the child is attached, as evidenced by at least three of the following:

   (1)   persistent and excessive worry about losing, or possible harm befalling, major attachment figures

   (2)   persistent and excessive worry that an untoward event will lead to separation from a major attachment figure (e.g., getting lost or being kidnapped)

   (3)   persistent reluctance or refusal to go to school or elsewhere because of fear of separation

   (4)   persistently and excessively scared or reluctant to be alone or without major attachment figures at home or without significant adults in other settings

   (5)   persistent reluctance or refusal to go to sleep without being near a major attachment figure or to sleep away from home

   (6)   repeated nightmares involving the theme of separation

   (7)   repeated complaints of physical symptoms (such as headaches, stomachaches, nausea, or vomiting) when separation from major attachment figures is anticipated or involved

   (8)   recurrent excessive distress when separation from home or major attachment figures is anticipated or involved

B.   Duration of the disturbance of at least four weeks.

C.   Onset before age 18.

D.   The disturbance causes clinically significant distress or impairment in social, academic (occupational), or other important areas of functioning.

E.   Does not occur exclusively during the course of a Pervasive Developmental Disorder, Schizophrenia, or other Psychotic Disorder.

Specify if: **early onset** if onset occurs before age 6

313.23 Selective Mutism (Elective Mutism)

A.   Consistent failure to speak in specific social situations (in which there is an expectation for speaking, e.g., at school) despite speaking in other situations.

B.   The disturbance interferes with educational or occupational achievement, or with social communication.

C.   Not better accounted for by a Communication Disorder (e.g., Stuttering) or by a lack of knowledge of the spoken language required in the social situation

D.   Duration of at least one month (not limited to the first month of school).

313.89 Reactive Attachment Disorder of Infancy or Early Childhood

A.   Markedly disturbed and developmentally inappropriate social relatedness in most contexts, beginning before age five, as evidenced by either (1) or (2):

(1)   persistent failure to initiate or respond in a developmentally appropriate fashion to most social interactions, as manifest by excessively inhibited, hypervigilant, or highly ambivalent and contradictory responses (e.g., the child may respond to caregivers with a mixture of approach, avoidance, and resistance to comforting, or may exhibit frozen watchfulness)

(2)   diffuse attachments as manifested by indiscriminate sociability with marked inability to exhibit appropriate selective attachments (e.g., excessive familiarity with relative strangers or lack of selectivity in choice of attachment figures).

B.   The disturbance in A is not accounted for solely by developmental delay (as in Mental Retardation) and is not a symptom of a Pervasive Developmental Disorder.

C.   Grossly pathogenic care as evidenced by at least one of the following:

(1)   persistent disregard of the child's basic emotional needs for comfort, stimulation, and affection.

(2)   persistent disregard of the child's basic physical needs

(3)   repeated changes of primary caregiver that prevent formation of stable attachments (e.g., frequent changes in foster care)

D.   There is a presumption that the care in C is responsible for the disturbed behavior in A (e.g., the disturbances in A began following the pathogenic care in C).

Specify type:
   Inhibited Type: if criterion A(1) predominates in the clinical presentation.
   Disinhibited Type: if criterion A(2) predominates in the clinical presentation.

307.3 Stereotypic Movement Disorder (Stereotypy/Habit Disorder)

A.   Repetitive, seemingly driven, and nonfunctional motor behavior (e.g., hand shaking or waving, body rocking, head banging, mouthing of objects, self-biting, picking at skin or bodily orifices, hitting own body).

B.   The behavior markedly interferes with normal activities or results in bodily injury to the individual that requires medical treatment (or would result in an injury if preventive measures were not used)

C.   If Mental Retardation or a Pervasive Developmental Disorder is present, the stereotypic or self-injurious behavior is of sufficient severity to become a focus of treatment.

D.   The behavior is not better accounted for by a compulsion (as in Obsessive-Compulsive Disorder) or a tic (as in Tic Disorder), and is not restricted to hair-pulling (as in Trichotillomania).

E.   The behaviors persist for four weeks or more.

Specify if **With Self-injurious Behavior**: if the behavior results in bodily damage that requires medical treatment (or would result in bodily damage if protective measures were not used).

313.9 Disorder of Infancy, Childhood, or Adolescence Not Otherwise Specified

This is a residual category for disorders with onset in infancy, childhood, or adolescence that do not meet criteria for any specific disorder in the classification.

Delirium, Dementia, Amnestic and Other Cognitive Disorders

Deliria

293.0 Delirium Due to a General Medical Condition

A. Disturbance of consciousness (i.e., reduced clarity of awareness of the environment) with reduced ability to focus, sustain, or shift attention.

B. Change in cognition (such as memory deficit, disorientation, language disturbance, perceptual disturbance) that is not better accounted for by a preexisting, established, or evolving dementia.

C. The disturbance develops over a short period of time (usually hours to days) and tends to fluctuate during the course of the day.

D. There is evidence from the history, physical examination, or laboratory findings of a general medical condition judged to be etiologically related to the disturbance.

Coding Note: if Delirium is superimposed on a pre-existing Dementia, indicate the Delirium by coding the appropriate subtype of the Dementia, e.g., 290.30 Dementia of the Alzheimer's Type, Late Onset, with delirium.

Substance-induced Delirium

A. Disturbance of consciousness (i.e., reduced clarity of awareness of the environment) with reduced ability to focus, sustain, or shift attention.

B. Change in cognition (such as memory deficit, disorientation, language disturbance, perceptual disturbance) that is not better accounted for by a preexisting, established, or evolving dementia.

C. The disturbance develops over a short period of time (usually hours to days) and tends to fluctuate during the course of the day.

D. There is evidence from the history, physical examination, or laboratory findings of substance (e.g., drugs of abuse, medication) intoxication or withdrawal judged to be etiologically related to the disturbance.

Code: (Specific Substance) Delirium
(291.0 Alcohol, 292.81 Amphetamine [or Related Substance], 292.81 Cannabis, 292.81 Cocaine, 292.81 Hallucinogen, 292.81 Inhalant, 292.81 Opioid, 292.81 Phencyclidine [or Related Substance], 292.81 Sedative, Hypnotic, or Anxiolytic, 292.81 Other [or Unknown] Substance [e.g., cimetidine, digitalis, benztropine])

Coding note: also code substance-specific Intoxication or Withdrawal if criteria are met).

Specify if: (see table on page xx for applicability by substance)
with onset during intoxication
with onset during withdrawal

Delirium Due to Multiple Etiologies

A.   Disturbance of consciousness (i.e., reduced clarity of awareness of the environment) with reduced ability to focus, sustain, or shift attention.

B.   Change in cognition (such as memory deficit, disorientation, language disturbance, perceptual disturbance) that is not better accounted for by a preexisting, established, or evolving dementia.

C.   The disturbance develops over a short period of time (usually hours to days) and tends to fluctuate during the course of the day.

D.   Evidence from the history, physical examination, or laboratory tests that the delirium has more than one etiology (e.g., more than one etiologic general medical condition, a general medical condition plus Substance Intoxication or medication side effect)

Coding Note: Use multiple codes reflecting specific Delirium and specific etiologies, e.g., 293.0 Delirium due to viral encephalitis, 292.81 Sedative-induced Delirium.

293.89 Delirium Not Otherwise Specified

Examples:

1)   a clinical presentation of delirium that is suspected to be due to a general medical condition or substance use but for which there is insufficient evidence to establish a specific etiologic relationship

2)   Delirium due to causes not listed above (e.g., sensory deprivation)

Dementias

Dementia of the Alzheimer's Type

A. The development of multiple cognitive deficits manifested by both:

    (1) memory impairment (inability to learn new information and to recall previously learned information)

    (2) at least one of the following cognitive disturbances:

        (a) aphasia (language disturbance)

        (b) apraxia (inability to carry out motor activities despite intact motor function)

        (c) agnosia (failure to recognize or identify objects despite intact sensory function)

        (d) disturbance in executive functioning (i.e., planning, organizing, sequencing, abstracting)

B. The course is characterized by gradual onset and continuing cognitive decline.

C. The cognitive deficits cause significant impairment in social or occupational functioning and represent a significant decline from a previous level of functioning.

D. The cognitive deficits in A are not due to any of the following:

    (1) central nervous system conditions that cause progressive deficits in memory and cognition (e.g., cerebrovascular disease, Parkinson's disease, Huntington's disease, subdural hematoma, normal pressure hydrocephalus)

    (2) systemic conditions that are known to cause dementia (e.g., hypothyroidism, vitamin B12 or folic acid deficiency, niacin deficiency, hypercalcemia, neurosyphilis, HIV infection)

    (3) Substance-induced conditions

E. The deficits do not occur exclusively during the course of Delirium.

F. Not better accounted for by another Axis I disorder (e.g., Major Depressive Disorder, Schizophrenia).

Code based on type of onset and predominant features:

With Early Onset: if onset at age 65 or below.
290.10 uncomplicated
290.11 with delirium
290.12 with delusions
290.13 with depressed mood
290.14 with hallucinations
290.15 with perceptual disturbance
290.16 with behavioral disturbance
290.17 with communication disturbance

With Late Onset: if onset after age 65.
290.00 uncomplicated
290.30 with delirium
290.20 with delusions
290.21 with depressed mood
290.22 with hallucinations
290.23 with perceptual disturbance
290.24 with behavioral disturbance
290.25 with communication disturbance

Coding Note: Also code 331.0 Alzheimer's Disease on Axis III

290.4x Vascular Dementia

A. The development of multiple cognitive deficits manifested by both:

   (1) memory impairment (inability to learn new information and to recall previously learned information)

   (2) at least one of the following cognitive disturbances:

      (a) aphasia (language disturbance)

      (b) apraxia (inability to carry out motor activities despite intact motor function)

      (c) agnosia (failure to recognize or identify objects despite intact sensory function)

      (d) disturbance in executive functioning (i.e., planning, organizing, sequencing, abstracting)

B.   Focal neurologic signs and symptoms (e.g., exaggeration of deep tendon reflexes, extensor plantar response, pseudobulbar palsy, gait abnormalities, weakness of an extremity) or laboratory evidence indicative of cerebral vascular disease (e.g., multiple infarctions involving cortex and underlying white matter) that are judged to be etiologically related to the disturbance.

C.   The cognitive deficits cause significant impairment in social or occupational functioning and represent a significant decline from a previous level of functioning.

D.   The deficits do not occur exclusively during the course of Delirium.

Code based on predominant features:
    290.40 uncomplicated
    290.41 with delirium
    290.42 with delusions
    290.43 with depressed mood
    290.44 with hallucinations
    290.45 with perceptual disturbance
    290.46 with behavioral disturbance
    290.47 with communication disturbance

Dementia Due to Other General Medical Conditions

A.   The development of multiple cognitive deficits manifested by both:

(1)   memory impairment (inability to learn new information and to recall previously learned information)

(2)   at least one of the following cognitive disturbances:

(a)   aphasia (language disturbance)

(b)   apraxia (inability to carry out motor activities despite intact motor function)

(c)   agnosia (failure to recognize or identify objects despite intact sensory function)

(d)   disturbance in executive functioning (i.e., planning, organizing, sequencing, abstracting)

B.   The cognitive deficits cause significant impairment in social or occupational functioning and represent a significant decline from a previous level of functioning.

C.   The deficits do not occur exclusively during the course of Delirium.

D.   There is evidence from the history, physical examination, or laboratory findings of one of the conditions listed below that is judged to be etiologically related to the disturbance.

294.9   Dementia Due to HIV Disease
Coding Note: Also code 043.1 HIV Disease on Axis III
294.1   Dementia Due to Head Trauma
Coding Note: Also code 905.0 Head Trauma on Axis III
294.1   Dementia Due to Parkinson's Disease
Coding Note: Also code 332.0 Parkinson's Disease on Axis III
294.1   Dementia Due to Huntington's Disease
Coding Note: Also code 333.4 Huntington's Disease on Axis III
290.10 Dementia Due to Pick's Disease
Coding Note: Also code 331.1 Pick's Disease on Axis III
290.10 Dementia Due to Creutzfeldt-Jakob Disease
Coding Note: Also code 046.1 Creutzfeldt-Jakob Disease on Axis III
294.1   Dementia Due to Other General Medical Condition (e.g., normal pressure hydrocephalus, hypothyroidism, brain tumor, vitamin B12 deficiency)

Substance-Induced Persisting Dementia

A.   The development of multiple cognitive deficits manifested by both:

   (1)   memory impairment (inability to learn new information and to recall previously learned information)

   (2)   at least one of the following cognitive disturbances:

      (a)   aphasia (language disturbance)

      (b)   apraxia (inability to carry out motor activities despite intact motor function)

      (c)   agnosia (failure to recognize or identify objects despite intact sensory function)

      (d)   disturbance in executive functioning (i.e., planning, organizing, sequencing, abstracting)

B.   The cognitive deficits cause significant impairment in social or occupational functioning and represent a significant decline from a previous level of functioning.

C.   The deficits do not occur exclusively during the course of Delirium.

D.   There is evidence from the history, physical examination, or laboratory findings of substance use (e.g., drugs of abuse, medication, toxin exposure) judged to be etiologically related to the disturbance.

Code: (Specific Substance) Persisting Dementia
(291.2 Alcohol, 292.82 Inhalant, 292.82 Sedative, Hypnotic, or Anxiolytic, 292.82 Other [or Unknown] Substance)

Dementia Due to Multiple Etiologies

A.   The development of multiple cognitive deficits manifested by both:

(1)   memory impairment (inability to learn new information and to recall previously learned information)

(2)   at least one of the following cognitive disturbances:

(a)   aphasia (language disturbance)

(b)   apraxia (inability to carry out motor activities despite intact motor function)

(c)   agnosia (failure to recognize or identify objects despite intact sensory function)

(d)   disturbance in executive functioning (i.e., planning, organizing, sequencing, abstracting)

B.   The cognitive deficits cause significant impairment in social or occupational functioning and represent a significant decline from a previous level of functioning.

C.   Evidence from the history, physical examination, or laboratory tests that the disturbance has more than one etiology (e.g., head trauma plus chronic alcohol use, Dementia of the Alzheimer's Type with the subsequent development of Vascular Dementia).

D.   The deficits do not occur exclusively during the course of Delirium.

Coding Note: Use multiple codes based on specific Dementias and specific etiologies, e.g., 290.00 Dementia of the Alzheimer's Type, 290.40 Vascular Dementia.

294.8 Dementia Not Otherwise Specified

Example: a clinical presentation of dementia for which there is insufficient evidence to establish a specific etiology.

Amnestic Disorders

294.0 Amnestic Disorder Due to a General Medical Condition

A. The development of memory impairment as manifested by the inability to learn new information **or** the inability to recall previously learned information.

B. The memory disturbance causes significant impairment in social or occupational functioning and represents a significant decline from a previous level of functioning.

C. The memory disturbance does not occur exclusively during the course of Delirium or Dementia.

D. There is evidence from the history, physical examination, or laboratory findings of a general medical condition (including physical trauma) judged to be etiologically related to the memory impairment.

Specify if:
   transient (if memory impairment lasts for one month or less)
   chronic (if memory impairment lasts for more than one month)

Substance-Induced Persisting Amnestic Disorder

A. The development of memory impairment as manifested by the inability to learn new information **or** the inability to recall previously learned information.

B. The memory disturbance causes significant impairment in social or occupational functioning and represents a significant decline from a previous level of functioning.

C. The memory disturbance does not occur exclusively during the course of Delirium or Dementia.

D. There is evidence from the history, physical examination, or laboratory findings of substance use (e.g., drugs of abuse, medication, toxin exposure) judged to be etiologically related to the disturbance.

Code: (Specific Substance) Persisting Amnestic Disorder
(291.1 Alcohol, 292.83 Sedative, Hypnotic, or Anxiolytic, 292.83 Other [or Unknown])

294.8 Amnestic Disorder Not Otherwise Specified

Example: a clinical presentation of amnestic disorder for which there is insufficient evidence to establish a specific etiology.

294.9 Cognitive Disorder Not Otherwise Specified

This category is for disorders characterized by cognitive dysfunction presumed to be due to either substance use or a general medical condition that do not meet criteria for any of the specific Deliria, Dementias, or Amnestic Disorders listed above, and that are not better classified as Delirium NOS, Dementia NOS, or Amnestic Disorder NOS. Example: Mild cognitive disorder, i.e., impairment in cognitive functioning as evidenced by neuropsychological testing or quantified clinical assessment, accompanied by objective evidence of a systemic illness or central nervous system dysfunction. (See page xx for suggested criteria).

Mental Disorders Due to a General Medical Condition

Text and criteria for the following disorders are included elsewhere (i.e., in the sections with which they share symptomatic presentations).

293.0 Delirium Due to a General Medical Condition
---.- Dementia Due to a General Medical Condition
294.0 Amnestic Disorder Due to a General Medical Condition
(in the Delirium, Dementia, Amnestic and Other Cognitive Disorders section, page xx)

293.8x Psychotic Disorder Due to a General Medical Condition (in the Schizophrenia and Other Psychotic Disorders section, page xx)

293.83 Mood Disorder Due to a General Medical Condition (in the Mood Disorders section, page xx)

293.89 Anxiety Disorder Due to a General Medical Condition (in the Anxiety Disorders section, page xx)

---.- Sexual Dysfunction Due to a General Medical Condition (in the Sexual Disorders section, page xx)

780.5x Sleep Disorder Due to a General Medical Condition (in the Sleep Disorders section, page xx)

293.89 Catatonic Disorder Due to a General Medical Condition

A. The presence of catatonia as manifested by motoric immobility; excessive motor activity (that is apparently purposeless and not influenced by external stimuli), extreme negativism, mutism, peculiarities of voluntary movement; echolalia, or echopraxia.

B. There is evidence from the history, physical examination, or laboratory findings of a general medical condition judged to be etiologically related to the catatonia.

C. The disturbance does not occur exclusively during the course of Delirium.

D. Not better accounted for by another mental disorder (e.g., manic episode).

310.1 Personality Change Due to a General Medical Condition

A.   A persistent personality disturbance that represents a change from the individual's previous characteristic personality pattern. (In children, a marked deviation from normal development or a significant change in the child's usual behavior patterns lasting at least one year).

B.   There is evidence from the history, physical examination, or laboratory findings of a general medical condition judged to be etiologically related to the personality change.

C.   The disturbance is not better accounted for by another mental disorder (including other Mental Disorders Due to a General Medical Condition)

D.   The disturbance causes clinically significant distress or impairment in social, occupational, or other important areas of functioning.

E.   The disturbance does not occur exclusively during Delirium and does not meet criteria for Dementia.

Specify **type:**

Labile Type: if the predominant feature is affective lability

Disinhibited Type: if the predominant feature is poor impulse control as evidenced by sexual indiscretions, etc.

Aggressive Type: if the predominant feature is aggressive behavior

Apathetic Type: if the predominant feature is marked apathy and indifference

Paranoid Type: if the predominant feature is suspiciousness or paranoid ideation

Other Type: for example, personality change associated with a seizure disorder

Combined Type: if more than one feature predominates in the clinical picture

Unspecified

293.9 Mental Disorder Not Otherwise Specified Due to a General Medical Condition

This residual category should be used for situations in which it has been established that the disturbance is due to a general medical condition, but the criteria are not met for a specific Mental Disorder Due to a General Medical Condition.   Examples include:

1) Postconcussional disorder: difficulty in memory or attention with associated symptoms following a head trauma. (see page xx for suggested criteria).

2) Dissociative symptoms due to complex partial seizures.

Substance-Related Disorders

DEPENDENCE AND ABUSE

Substance Dependence

A maladaptive pattern of substance use, leading to clinically significant impairment or distress, as manifested by three or more of the following occurring at any time in the same twelve month period:

(1)   tolerance, as defined by either of the following:

    (a)   need for markedly increased amounts of the substance to achieve intoxication or desired effect

    (b)   markedly diminished effect with continued use of the same amount of the substance

(2)   withdrawal, as manifested by either of the following:

    (a)   the characteristic Withdrawal syndrome for the substance (refer to criteria A and B of the criteria sets for Withdrawal from the specific substances)

    (b)   the same (or closely related) substance is taken to relieve or avoid withdrawal symptoms

(3)   the substance is often taken in larger amounts or over a longer period than was intended

(4)   a persistent desire or unsuccessful efforts to cut down or control substance use

(5)   a great deal of time is spent in activities necessary to obtain the substance (e.g., visiting multiple doctors or driving long distances), use the substance (e.g., chain-smoking), or recover from its effects

(6)   important social, occupational, or recreational activities given up or reduced because of substance use

(7)   continued substance use despite knowledge of having had a persistent or recurrent physical or psychological problem that was likely to have been caused or exacerbated by the substance (e.g., current cocaine use despite recognition of cocaine-induced depression, or continued drinking despite recognition that an ulcer was made worse by alcohol consumption)

Specify if:
> **With Physiological Dependence:** Evidence of tolerance or withdrawal (i.e., either item (1) or (2) is present).
> **Without Physiological Dependence:** No evidence of tolerance or withdrawal (i.e., neither item (1) nor (2) is present).

Course Modifiers

These course modifiers apply only to dependence. Insufficient data are available on the course of abuse. Although criteria for abuse are separate from those for dependence, abuse and dependence are hierarchical, i.e., once an individual has ever had a pattern of substance use which meets criteria for dependence, the person can no longer qualify for a diagnosis of abuse for that substance. Thus, when determining whether an individual is in partial or full remission from dependence, the clinician must consider substance use behavior covered in the criteria sets for both Substance Dependence and Substance Abuse.

Remission: A person is not classified as being in remission until he or she has not experienced any of the criterion items for dependence or abuse for at least one month.

Early Remission. The first twelve months following cessation of problems with the substance is a period of particularly high risk for relapse, thus it is given a special designation: Early Remission. There are two categories:

> **Early Full Remission:** No criteria for dependence or abuse have been met for the last one to twelve months.

> **Early Partial Remission:** Full criteria for dependence have not been met for the last one to twelve months; however at least one of the criteria for dependence or abuse have been met, intermittently or continuously, during this period of Early Remission.

Sustained Remission. When twelve months of Early Remission have passed, the person is in Sustained Remission. There are two categories:

> **Sustained Full Remission:** None of the criteria for dependence or abuse have been met at any time during the prior twelve months or longer.

> **Sustained Partial Remission:** Full criteria for dependence have not been met for a period of twelve months or longer; however, at least one of criteria for dependence or abuse have been met, intermittently or continuously, during this period of Sustained Remission.

Note: The differentiation of "Sustained Full Remission" from recovered (no current substance use disorder) requires consideration of the length of time since the last period of disturbance, the total duration of the disturbance, and the need for continued evaluation.

The following modifiers apply so long as the person is being treated with agonist therapy or is in a controlled environment:

On Agonist Therapy: On a prescribed supervised agonist medication related to the substance and the criteria for dependence or abuse (other than tolerance or withdrawal) have not been met for the agonist medication in the past month. This category also applies to those being treated for dependence using a mixed agonist/antagonist having prominent agonist properties.

In A Controlled Environment: No criteria for dependence or abuse are met but the person is in an environment for one month or longer where controlled substances are highly restricted. Examples are closely-supervised and substance-free jails, therapeutic communities, or locked hospital units. Occasionally persons will be on agonist therapy while also in a controlled environment. In such cases, both course modifiers apply.

Note: Just as the remission categories require a transitional month during which no criteria for dependence or abuse are met, the one month period after cessation of agonist therapy or release from a controlled environment is a corresponding transition period. Thus, persons in this one month period are still considered dependent. They can move into a remission category after no dependence or abuse criteria are met for one month.

Substance Abuse

A. A maladaptive pattern of substance use leading to clinically significant impairment or distress, as manifested by one or more of the following occurring at any time during the same twelve month period:

   (1) recurrent substance use resulting in a failure to fulfill major role obligations at work, school, or home (e.g., repeated absences or poor work performance related to substance use; substance-related absences, suspensions, or expulsions from school; neglect of children or household)

   (2) recurrent substance use in situations in which it is physically hazardous (e.g., driving an automobile or operating a machine when impaired by substance use)

   (3) recurrent substance-related legal problems (e.g., arrests for substance-related disorderly conduct)

   (4) continued substance use despite having persistent or recurrent social or interpersonal problems caused or exacerbated by the effects of the substance (e.g., arguments with spouse about consequences of intoxication, physical fights)

B. Has never met the criteria for Substance Dependence for this class of substance.

Substance Intoxication

A.　The development of a reversible substance-specific syndrome due to recent ingestion of (or exposure to) a substance. (Note: different substances may produce similar or identical syndromes).

B.　Clinically significant maladaptive behavioral or psychological changes due to the effect of the substance on the central nervous system (e.g., belligerence, mood lability, cognitive impairment, impaired judgment, impaired social or occupational functioning) developing during or shortly after use of the substance.

C.　Not due to a general medical condition and not better accounted for by another mental disorder.

Substance Withdrawal

A.　The development of a substance-specific syndrome due to the cessation of, or reduction in, the intake of a substance that the person previously used regularly.

B.　The substance-specific syndrome causes clinically significant distress or impairment in social, occupational, or other important areas of functioning.

C.　Not due to a general medical condition and not better accounted for by another mental disorder.

MAJOR SUBSTANCE DIAGNOSES

Substance	Intoxication	Withdrawal	Persisting	Abuse	Dependence
Alcohol	X	X	X	X	X
Amphetamine	X	X		X	X
Caffeine	X				
Cannabis	X			X	X
Cocaine	X	X		X	X
Hallucinogen	X		X	X	X
Inhalant	X		X	X	X
Nicotine		X			X
Opioid	X	X		X	X
Phencyclidine	X			X	X
Sed-Hyp-Anxiolyic	X	X	X	X	X
Other or Unspecified	X	X	X	X	X

TABLE OF SUBSTANCE-INDUCED DISORDERS DISTRIBUTED IN OTHER SECTIONS WITH PHENOMENOLOGICALLY SIMILAR DISORDERS

	Delirium	Dementia	Amnestic	Psychotic	Mood	Anxiety	Sex	Sleep
Alcohol	I/W	P	P	I/W	I/W	I/W	I	I/W
Amphetamine	I			I	I/W	I	I	I/W
Caffeine						I		I
Cannabis	I			I		I		
Cocaine	I			I	I/W	I	I	I/W
Hallucinogen	I			I*	I	I		
Inhalant	I	P		I	I	I		
Nicotine								
Opioid	I			I		I	I	I/W
PCP	I			I	I	I		
Sedative	I/W	P	P	I/W	I/W	W	I	I/W
Other	I/W	P	P	I/W	I/W	I/W	I	I/W

*also Hallucinogen Persisting Perception Disorder (Flashbacks)

Note: I, W, I/W, or P in the table indicates that the category is recognized in DSM-IV. In addition, "I" indicates that the modifier "with onset during intoxication" may be noted for the category; "W" indicates that the modifier "with onset during withdrawal" may be noted for the category; "I/W" indicates that either "with onset during intoxication" or "with onset during withdrawal" may be noted for the category; "P" indicates the disorder is "persisting," i.e., the disturbance persists long after the acute effects of intoxication and withdrawal.

SPECIFIC SUBSTANCE-RELATED DISORDERS

Alcohol Use Disorders

303.90 Alcohol Dependence (see page xx)
305.00 Alcohol Abuse (see page xx)

303.00 Alcohol Intoxication

A. Recent ingestion of alcohol in an amount that is sufficient to cause intoxication in most people.

B. Clinically significant maladaptive behavioral or psychological changes (e.g., inappropriate sexual or aggressive behavior, mood lability, impaired judgment, impaired social or occupational functioning) developing during, or shortly after, alcohol ingestion.

C. At least one of the following signs, developing during or shortly after use:

    (1) slurred speech
    (2) incoordination
    (3) unsteady gait
    (4) nystagmus
    (5) impairment in attention or memory
    (6) stupor or coma

D. Not due to a general medical condition and not better accounted for by another mental disorder.

291.8 Alcohol Withdrawal

A. Cessation (or reduction) of alcohol use which has been heavy and prolonged.

B. At least two of the following, developing within several hours to a few days after A:

    (1) autonomic hyperactivity (e.g., sweating or pulse rate greater than 100)
    (2) increased hand tremor
    (3) insomnia
    (4) nausea or vomiting
    (5) transient visual, tactile, or auditory hallucinations or illusions
    (6) psychomotor agitation
    (7) anxiety
    (8) grand mal seizures

C. The symptoms in B cause clinically significant distress or impairment in social, occupational, or other important areas of functioning.

D.   Not due to a general medical condition and not better accounted for by another mental disorder.

Specify if **with perceptual disturbances:** auditory, visual, or tactile illusions; altered perceptions, or hallucinations with intact reality testing.

291.0 Alcohol Delirium (see page xx)
> *Specify if*:
> > with onset during intoxication
> > with onset during withdrawal

291.2 Alcohol Persisting Dementia (see page xx)

291.1 Alcohol Persisting Amnestic Disorder (see page xx)

291.5 Alcohol Psychotic Disorder, with delusions (see page xx)
> *Specify if*:
> > with onset during intoxication
> > with onset during withdrawal

291.3 Alcohol Psychotic Disorder, with hallucinations (see page xx)
> *Specify if*:
> > with onset during intoxication
> > with onset during withdrawal

291.8 Alcohol Mood Disorder (see page xx)
> *Specify if*:
> > with onset during intoxication
> > with onset during withdrawal

291.8 Alcohol Anxiety Disorder (see page xx)
> *Specify if*:
> > with onset during intoxication
> > with onset during withdrawal

292.8 Alcohol Sexual Dysfunction (see page xx)
> *Specify if*:
> > with onset during intoxication

292.89 Alcohol Sleep Disorder (see page xx)
> *Specify if*:
> > with onset during intoxication
> > with onset during withdrawal

291.9 Alcohol Use Disorder Not Otherwise Specified

This category is for disorders associated with use of alcohol that are not classifiable as Alcohol Dependence, Alcohol Abuse, Alcohol Intoxication, Alcohol Withdrawal, Alcohol Delirium, Alcohol Persisting Dementia, Alcohol Persisting Amnestic Disorder, Alcohol Psychotic Disorder, Alcohol Mood Disorder, Alcohol Anxiety Disorder, or Alcohol Sexual Dysfunction and Alcohol Sleep Disorder.

Example: Idiosyncratic Alcohol Intoxication, i.e., maladaptive behavioral changes occurring within minutes of ingesting an amount of alcohol insufficient to induce intoxication in most people.

Amphetamine (or Related Substance) Use Disorders

304.40 Amphetamine (or Related Substance) Dependence (see page xx)
305.70 Amphetamine (or Related Substance) Abuse (see page xx)

305.70 Amphetamine (or Related Substance) Intoxication

A. Recent use of amphetamine or a related substance (e.g., methylphenidate).

B. Clinically significant maladaptive behavioral or psychological changes (e.g., euphoria or affective blunting; changes in sociability; hypervigilance; interpersonal sensitivity; anxiety, tension, or anger; stereotyped behaviors; impaired judgment; or impaired social or occupational functioning) developing during, or shortly after, use of amphetamine or a related substance.

C. At least two of the following, developing during, or shortly after, use:

    (1) tachycardia or bradycardia
    (2) pupillary dilation
    (3) elevated or lowered blood pressure
    (4) perspiration or chills
    (5) nausea or vomiting
    (6) evidence of weight loss
    (7) psychomotor agitation or retardation
    (8) muscular weakness, respiratory depression, chest pain, or cardiac arrhythmias
    (9) confusion, seizures, dyskinesias, dystonias, or coma

D. Not due to a general medical condition and not better accounted for by another mental disorder.

Specify if **with perceptual disturbances:** auditory, visual, or tactile illusions; altered perceptions, or hallucinations with intact reality testing.

292.0 Amphetamine (or Related Substance) Withdrawal

A. Cessation (or reduction) of amphetamine (or related substance) use which has been heavy and prolonged.

B. Dysphoric mood and at least two of the following physiological changes, developing within a few hours to several days after A:

    (1) fatigue
    (2) vivid, unpleasant dreams
    (3) insomnia or hypersomnia
    (4) increased appetite
    (5) psychomotor retardation or agitation

C. The symptoms in B cause clinically significant distress or impairment in social, occupational, or other important areas of functioning.

D. Not due to a general medical condition and not better accounted for by another mental disorder.

292.81 Amphetamine (or Related Substance) Delirium (see page xx)
Specify if:
    with onset during intoxication
291.11 Amphetamine (or Related Substance) Psychotic Disorder, with delusions (see page xx)
Specify if:
    with onset during intoxication
291.1 Amphetamine (or Related Substance) Psychotic Disorder, with hallucinations (see page xx)
Specify if:
    with onset during intoxication
292.8 Amphetamine (or Related Substance) Mood Disorder (see page xx)
Specify if:
    with onset during intoxication
    with onset during withdrawal
292.89 Amphetamine (or Related Substance) Anxiety Disorder (see page xx)
Specify if:
    with onset during intoxication
292.89 Amphetamine (or Related Substance) Sexual Dysfunction (see page xx)
Specify if:
    with onset during intoxication
292.89 Amphetamine (or Related Substance) Sleep Disorder (see page xx)
Specify if:
    with onset during intoxication
    with onset during withdrawal

292.9 Amphetamine (or Related Substance) Use Disorder Not Otherwise Specified

This category is for disorders associated with use of amphetamine (or a related substance) that are not classifiable as Amphetamine Dependence, Amphetamine Abuse, Amphetamine Intoxication, Amphetamine Withdrawal, Amphetamine Delirium, Amphetamine Psychotic Disorder, Amphetamine Mood Disorder, Amphetamine Anxiety Disorder, Amphetamine Sexual Dysfunction, or Amphetamine Sleep Disorder.

Caffeine Use Disorders

305.90 Caffeine Intoxication

A. Recent consumption of caffeine, usually in excess of 250 mg. (e.g., more than 2-3 cups of brewed coffee).

B. At least five of the following signs, developing during, or shortly after, caffeine use:

    (1) restlessness
    (2) nervousness
    (3) excitement
    (4) insomnia
    (5) flushed face
    (6) diuresis
    (7) gastrointestinal disturbance
    (8) muscle twitching
    (9) rambling flow of thought and speech
    (10) tachycardia or cardiac arrhythmia
    (11) periods of inexhaustibility
    (12) psychomotor agitation

C. The symptoms in B cause clinically significant distress or impairment in social, occupational, or other important areas of functioning.

D. Not due to a general medical condition and not better accounted for by another mental disorder, such as an Anxiety Disorder.

292.84 Caffeine Anxiety Disorder (see page xx)
Specify if:
    with onset during intoxication
292.89 Caffeine Sleep Disorder (see page xx)
Specify if:
    with onset during intoxication

292.9 Caffeine Use Disorder Not Otherwise Specified

This category is for disorders associated with use of caffeine that are not classifiable as Caffeine Intoxication, Caffeine Anxiety Disorder or Caffeine Sleep Disorder. Example: Caffeine Withdrawal (see page xx for suggested criteria).

Cannabis Use Disorders

304.30 Cannabis Dependence (see page xx)
305.20 Cannabis Abuse (see page xx)

305.20 Cannabis Intoxication

A.   Recent use of cannabis.

B.   Clinically significant maladaptive behavioral or psychological changes (e.g., impaired motor coordination, euphoria, anxiety, sensation of slowed time, impaired judgment, social withdrawal) developing during, or shortly after, cannabis use.

C.   At least two of the following signs, developing within two hours of cannabis use:

   (1)   conjunctival injection
   (2)   increased appetite
   (3)   dry mouth
   (4)   tachycardia

D.   Not due to a general medical condition and not better accounted for by another mental disorder.

Specify if **with perceptual disturbances:** auditory, visual, or tactile illusions; altered perceptions, or hallucinations with intact reality testing.

292.81 Cannabis Delirium (see page xx)
   Specify if:
      with onset during intoxication
291.11 Cannabis Psychotic Disorder, with Delusions (see page xx)
   Specify if:
      with onset during intoxication
292.89 Cannabis Anxiety Disorder (see page xx)
   Specify if:
      with onset during intoxication

292.9 Cannabis Use Disorder Not Otherwise Specified

This category is for disorders associated with use of cannabis that are not classifiable as Cannabis Dependence, Cannabis Abuse, Cannabis Intoxication, Cannabis Delirium, Cannabis Psychotic Disorder, or Cannabis Anxiety Disorder.

Cocaine Use Disorders

304.20 Cocaine Dependence (see page xx)
305.60 Cocaine Abuse (see page xx)

305.60 Cocaine Intoxication

A.   Recent use of cocaine.

B.   Clinically significant maladaptive behavioral or psychological changes (e.g., euphoria or affective blunting; changes in sociability; hypervigilance; interpersonal sensitivity; anxiety, tension, or anger; stereotyped behaviors; impaired judgment; or impaired social or occupational functioning) developing during, or shortly after, use of cocaine.

C.   At least two of the following, developing during, or shortly after, use:

(1)   tachycardia or bradycardia
(2)   pupillary dilation
(3)   elevated or lowered blood pressure
(4)   perspiration or chills
(5)   nausea or vomiting
(6)   evidence of weight loss
(7)   psychomotor agitation or retardation
(8)   muscular weakness, respiratory depression, chest pain, or cardiac arrhythmias
(9)   confusion, seizures, dyskinesias, dystonias, or coma

D.   Not due to a general medical condition and not better accounted for by another mental disorder.

Specify if **with perceptual disturbances:** auditory, visual, or tactile illusions; altered perceptions, or hallucinations with intact reality testing.

292.0 Cocaine Withdrawal

A.   Cessation (or reduction) of cocaine use which has been heavy and prolonged.

B.   Dysphoric mood and at least two of the following physiological changes, developing within a few hours to several days after A:

(1)   fatigue
(2)   vivid, unpleasant dreams
(3)   insomnia or hypersomnia
(4)   increased appetite
(5)   psychomotor retardation or agitation

C.   The symptoms in B cause clinically significant distress or impairment in social, occupational, or other important areas of functioning.

D.   Not due to a general medical condition and not better accounted for by another mental disorder.

292.81 Cocaine Delirium (see page xx)
Specify if:
    with onset during intoxication
291.11 Cocaine Psychotic Disorder, with delusions (see page xx)
Specify if:
    with onset during intoxication
291.12 Cocaine Psychotic Disorder, with hallucinations (see page xx)
Specify if:
    with onset during intoxication
292.84 Cocaine Mood Disorder (see page xx)
Specify if:
    with onset during intoxication
    with onset during withdrawal
292.89 Cocaine Anxiety Disorder (see page xx)
Specify if:
    with onset during intoxication
292.89 Cocaine Sexual Dysfunction (see page xx)
Specify if:
    with onset during intoxication
292.89 Cocaine Sleep Disorder (see page xx)
Specify if:
    with onset during intoxication
    with onset during withdrawal

292.9 Cocaine Use Disorder Not Otherwise Specified

This category is for disorders associated with use of cocaine that are not classifiable as Cocaine Dependence, Cocaine Abuse, Cocaine Intoxication, Cocaine Withdrawal, Cocaine Delirium, Cocaine Psychotic Disorder, Cocaine Mood Disorder, Cocaine Anxiety Disorder, Cocaine Sexual Dysfunction or Cocaine Sleep Disorder.

Hallucinogen Use Disorders

304.50 Hallucinogen Dependence (see page xx)
305.30 Hallucinogen Abuse (see page xx)

305.30 Hallucinogen Intoxication

A.   Recent use of a hallucinogen.

B.   Clinically significant maladaptive behavioral or psychological changes (e.g., marked anxiety or depression; ideas of reference; fear of losing one's mind; paranoid ideation, impaired judgment; or impaired social or occupational functioning) developing during, or shortly after, hallucinogen use.

C.   Perceptual changes occurring in a state of full wakefulness and alertness (e.g., subjective intensification of perceptions, depersonalization, derealization, illusions, hallucinations, synesthesias) developing during, or shortly after, hallucinogen use.

D.   At least two of the following signs, developing during, or shortly after, use:

   (1)   pupillary dilation
   (2)   tachycardia
   (3)   sweating
   (4)   palpitations
   (5)   blurring of vision
   (6)   tremors
   (7)   incoordination

E.   Not due to a general medical condition and not better accounted for by another mental disorder.

292.89 Hallucinogen Persisting Perception Disorder (Flashbacks)

A. The reexperiencing, following cessation of use of a hallucinogen, of one or more of the perceptual symptoms that were experienced while intoxicated with the hallucinogen (e.g., geometric hallucinations, false perceptions of movement in the peripheral visual fields, flashes of color, intensified colors, trails of images of moving objects, positive afterimages, halos around objects, macropsia, and micropsia).

B. The symptoms in A cause clinically significant distress or impairment in social, occupational, or other important areas of functioning.

C. Not due to a general medical condition (e.g., anatomic lesions and infections of the brain, visual epilepsies) and not better accounted for by another mental disorder (e.g., Delirium, Dementia, Schizophrenia), entopic imagery, or hypnopompic hallucinations.

292.81 Hallucinogen Delirium (see page xx)
Specify if:
> with onset during intoxication

291.11 Hallucinogen Psychotic Disorder, with delusions (see page xx)
Specify if:
> with onset during intoxication

291.12 Hallucinogen Psychotic Disorder, with hallucinations (see page xx)
Specify if:
> with onset during intoxication

292.84 Hallucinogen Mood Disorder (see page xx)
Specify if:
> with onset during intoxication

292.89 Hallucinogen Anxiety Disorder (see page xx)
Specify if:
> with onset during intoxication

292.9 Hallucinogen Use Disorder Not Otherwise Specified

This category is for disorders associated with use of hallucinogens that are not classifiable as Hallucinogen Dependence, Hallucinogen Abuse, Hallucinogen Intoxication, Hallucinogen Delirium, Hallucinogen Psychotic Disorder, Hallucinogen Mood Disorder, Hallucinogen Anxiety Disorder or Hallucinogen Persisting Perception Disorder.

Inhalant Use Disorders

304.60 Inhalant Dependence (see page xx)
305.90 Inhalant Abuse (see page xx)

305.90 Inhalant Intoxication

A. Recent intentional use or short-term, high-dose exposure to volatile inhalants (excluding anesthetic gases and short-acting vasodilators).

B. Clinically significant maladaptive behavioral or psychological changes (e.g., belligerence, assaultiveness, apathy, impaired judgment, impaired social or occupational functioning) developing during, or shortly after the use of, or exposure to, volatile inhalants.

C. At least two of the following signs, developing during, or shortly after, use or exposure:

    (1) dizziness
    (2) nystagmus
    (3) incoordination
    (4) slurred speech
    (5) unsteady gait
    (6) lethargy
    (7) depressed reflexes
    (8) psychomotor retardation
    (9) tremor
    (10) generalized muscle weakness
    (11) blurred vision or diplopia
    (12) stupor or coma
    (13) euphoria

D. Not due to a general medical condition and not better accounted for by another mental disorder.

292.81 Inhalant Delirium (see page xx)
Specify if:
    with onset during intoxication
292.82 Inhalant Persisting Dementia (see page xx)
291.11 Inhalant Psychotic Disorder, with delusions (see page xx)
Specify if:
    with onset during intoxication
291.12 Inhalant Psychotic Disorder, with hallucinations (see page xx)
Specify if:
    with onset during intoxication

292.84 Inhalant Mood Disorder (see page xx)
    Specify if:
        with onset during intoxication
292.89 Inhalant Anxiety Disorder (see page xx)
    Specify if:
        with onset during intoxication

292.9 Inhalant Use Disorder Not Otherwise Specified

This category is for disorders associated with use of inhalants that are not classifiable as Inhalant Dependence, Inhalant Abuse, Inhalant Intoxication, Inhalant Delirium, Inhalant Persisting Dementia, Inhalant Mood Disorder or Inhalant Anxiety Disorder.

Nicotine Use Disorders

305.10 Nicotine Dependence (see page xx)

292.0 Nicotine Withdrawal

A.   Daily use of nicotine for at least several weeks.

B.   Abrupt cessation of nicotine use, or reduction in the amount of nicotine used, followed within 24 hours by at least four of the following signs:

    (1)   dysphoric or depressed mood
    (2)   insomnia
    (3)   irritability, frustration, or anger
    (4)   anxiety
    (5)   difficulty concentrating
    (6)   restlessness
    (7)   decreased heart rate
    (8)   increased appetite or weight gain

C.   The symptoms in B cause clinically significant distress or impairment in social, occupational, or other important areas of functioning.

D.   Not due to a general medical condition and not better accounted for by another mental disorder.

292.9 Nicotine Use Disorder Not Otherwise Specified

This category is for disorders associated with use of Nicotine that are not classifiable as Nicotine Dependence or Nicotine Withdrawal.

Opioid Use Disorders

304.00 Opioid Dependence (see page xx)
305.50 Opioid Abuse (see page xx)

305.50 Opioid Intoxication

A. Recent use of an opioid.

B. Clinically significant maladaptive behavioral or psychological changes (e.g., initial euphoria followed by apathy, dysphoria, psychomotor agitation or retardation, impaired judgment, or impaired social or occupational functioning) developing during, or shortly after, opioid use.

C. Pupillary constriction (or pupillary dilation due to anoxia from severe overdose) and at least one of the following signs, developing during, or shortly after, opioid use:

    (1) drowsiness or coma
    (2) slurred speech
    (3) impairment in attention or memory

D. Not due to a general medical condition and not better accounted for by another mental disorder.

Specify if **with perceptual disturbances:** auditory, visual, or tactile illusions; altered perceptions, or hallucinations with intact reality testing.

292.0 Opioid Withdrawal

A. Either of the following:

    (1) Cessation (or reduction) of opioid use which has been heavy and prolonged (several weeks or longer).

    (2) Administration of an opioid antagonist after a period of opioid use

B. At least three of the following, developing within minutes to several days after A:

    (1) dysphoric mood
    (2) nausea or vomiting
    (3) muscle aches
    (4) lacrimation or rhinorrhea
    (5) pupillary dilation, piloerection, or sweating
    (6) diarrhea
    (7) yawning
    (8) fever
    (9) insomnia

C. The symptoms in B cause clinically significant distress or impairment in social, occupational, or other important areas of functioning.

D. Not due to a general medical condition and not better accounted for by another mental disorder.

292.81 Opioid Delirium (see page xx)
Specify if:
    with onset during intoxication
291.11 Opioid Psychotic Disorder, with delusions (see page xx)
Specify if:
    with onset during intoxication
291.12 Opioid Psychotic Disorder, with hallucinations (see page xx)
Specify if:
    with onset during intoxication
292.84 Opioid Mood Disorder (see page xx)
Specify if:
    with onset during intoxication
292.89 Opioid Sleep Disorder (see page xx)
Specify if:
    with onset during intoxication
    with onset during withdrawal
292.89 Opioid Sexual Dysfunction (see page xx)
Specify if:
    with onset during intoxication

292.9 Opioid Use Disorder Not Otherwise Specified

This category is for disorders associated with use of opioids that are not classifiable as Opioid Dependence, Opioid Abuse, Opioid Intoxication, Opioid Withdrawal, Opioid Delirium, Opioid Psychotic Disorder, Opioid Mood Disorder, Opioid Sexual Dysfunction or Opioid Sleep Disorder.

Phencyclidine (or Related Substance) Use Disorders

304.90 Phencyclidine (or Related Substance) Dependence (see page xx)
305.90 Phencyclidine (or Related Substance) Abuse (see page xx)

305.90 Phencyclidine (or Related Substance) Intoxication

A.   Recent use of phencyclidine (or a related substance).

B.   Clinically significant maladaptive behavioral changes (e.g., belligerence, assaultiveness, impulsiveness, unpredictability, psychomotor agitation, impaired judgment, or impaired social or occupational functioning) developing during, or shortly after, use of phencyclidine.

C.   Within an hour (less when smoked, "snorted," or used intravenously), at least two of the following signs:

    (1)   vertical or horizontal nystagmus
    (2)   hypertension or tachycardia
    (3)   numbness or diminished responsiveness to pain
    (4)   ataxia
    (5)   dysarthria
    (6)   muscle rigidity
    (7)   seizures or coma
    (8)   hyperacusis

D.   Not due to a general medical condition and not better accounted for by another mental disorder.

Specify if **with perceptual disturbances:** auditory, visual, or tactile illusions; altered perceptions, or hallucinations with intact reality testing.

292.81 Phencyclidine (or Related Substance) Delirium (see page xx)
    Specify if:
        with onset during intoxication
291.11 Phencyclidine (or Related Substance) Psychotic Disorder, with delusions (see page xx)
    Specify if:
        with onset during intoxication
291.12 Phencyclidine (or Related Substance) Psychotic Disorder, with hallucinations (see page xx)
    Specify if:
        with onset during intoxication
292.84 Phencyclidine (or Related Substance) Mood Disorder (see page xx)
    Specify if:
        with onset during intoxication
292.89 Phencyclidine (or Related Substance) Anxiety Disorder (see page xx)
    Specify if:
        with onset during intoxication

292.9 Phencyclidine (or Related Substance) Use Disorder Not Otherwise Specified

This category is for disorders associated with use of phencyclidine that are not classifiable as Phencyclidine Dependence, Phencyclidine Abuse, Phencyclidine Intoxication, Phencyclidine Delirium, Phencyclidine Psychotic Disorder, Phencyclidine Mood Disorder, and Phencyclidine Anxiety Disorder.

Sedative, Hypnotic, or Anxiolytic Substance Use Disorders

304.10 Sedative, Hypnotic, or Anxiolytic Dependence (see page xx)
305.40 Sedative, Hypnotic, or Anxiolytic Abuse (see page xx)

305.40 Sedative, Hypnotic, or Anxiolytic Intoxication

A.   Recent use of a sedative, hypnotic, or anxiolytic.

B.   Clinically significant maladaptive behavioral or psychological changes (e.g., inappropriate sexual or aggressive behavior, mood lability, impaired judgment, impaired social or occupational functioning) developing during, or shortly after, use of a sedative, hypnotic, or anxiolytic.

C.   At least one of the following signs, developing during, or shortly after, use:

    (1)   slurred speech
    (2)   incoordination
    (3)   unsteady gait
    (4)   nystagmus
    (5)   impairment in attention or memory
    (6)   stupor or coma

D.   Not due to a general medical condition and not better accounted for by another mental disorder.

292.0 Sedative, Hypnotic, or Anxiolytic Withdrawal

A.   Cessation (or reduction) of sedative, hypnotic, or anxiolytic use, which has been heavy and prolonged.

B.   At least two of the following, developing within several hours to a few days after A:

    (1)   autonomic hyperactivity (e.g., sweating or pulse rate greater than 100)
    (2)   increased hand tremor
    (3)   insomnia
    (4)   nausea or vomiting
    (5)   transient visual, tactile, or auditory hallucinations or illusions
    (6)   psychomotor agitation
    (7)   anxiety
    (8)   grand mal seizures

C.   The symptoms in B cause clinically significant distress or impairment in social, occupational, or other important areas of functioning.

D.   Not due to a general medical condition and not better accounted for by another mental disorder.

Specify if **with perceptual disturbances:** auditory, visual, or tactile illusions; altered perceptions, or hallucinations with intact reality testing.

292.81 Sedative, Hypnotic, or Anxiolytic Delirium (see page xx)
Specify if:
    with onset during intoxication
    with onset during withdrawal
292.82 Sedative, Hypnotic, or Anxiolytic Persisting Dementia (see page xx)
292.83 Sedative, Hypnotic, or Anxiolytic Persisting Amnestic Disorder (see page xx)
291.11 Sedative, Hypnotic or Anxiolytic Psychotic Disorder, with delusions (see page xx)
Specify if:
    with onset during intoxication
    with onset during withdrawal
291.12 Sedative, Hypnotic or Anxiolytic Psychotic Disorder, with hallucinations (see page xx)
Specify if:
    with onset during intoxication
    with onset during withdrawal
292.84 Sedative, Hypnotic, or Anxiolytic Mood Disorder (see page xx)
Specify if:
    with onset during intoxication
    with onset during withdrawal

292.89 Sedative, Hypnotic, or Anxiolytic Anxiety Disorder (see page xx)
  Specify if:
    with onset during withdrawal
?292.89 Sedative, Hypnotic, or Anxiolytic Sleep Disorder (see page xx)
  Specify if:
    with onset during intoxication
    with onset during withdrawal
?292.89 Sedative, Hypnotic, or Anxiolytic Sexual Dysfunction (see page xx)
  Specify if:
    with onset during intoxication

292.9 Sedative, Hypnotic, or Anxiolytic Use Disorder Not Otherwise Specified

This category is for disorders associated with use of sedatives, hypnotics, or anxiolytics that are not classifiable as Sedative, Hypnotic or Anxiolytic Dependence; Sedative, Hypnotic or Anxiolytic Abuse; Sedative, Hypnotic or Anxiolytic Intoxication; Sedative, Hypnotic or Anxiolytic Withdrawal; Sedative, Hypnotic, or Anxiolytic Delirium; Sedative, Hypnotic or Anxiolytic Psychotic Disorder; Sedative, Hypnotic, or Anxiolytic Mood Disorder; Sedative, Hypnotic, or Anxiolytic Anxiety Disorder; Sedative, Hypnotic, or Anxiolytic Sexual Dysfunction; or Sedative, Hypnotic, or Anxiolytic Sleep Disorder.

Polysubstance Use Disorder

304.80 Polysubstance Dependence

This category should be used when, for a period of six months, the person has repeatedly used at least three categories of substances (not including nicotine and caffeine), but no single substance has predominated. During this period, the criteria have been met for Substance Dependence for the substances considered as a group, but not for any single specific substance.

Other (or Unknown) Substance Use Disorders

This group of disorders is for classifying substance-induced conditions associated with substances not listed above. Examples include anabolic steroids, nitrite inhalants ("poppers"), nitrous oxide, over-the-counter and prescription medications (e.g., cortisol, cimetidine, digitalis, benztropine), and other substances that have psychoactive effects. In addition, these categories may be used when the specific substance is unknown (e.g., an intoxication after taking a bottle of unlabeled pills).

Anabolic steroids. These drugs sometimes produce an initial sense of enhanced well-being (or even euphoria), which is replaced after repeated use by lack of energy, irritability, and other forms of dysphoria. Continued use of these substances may lead to more serious psychological problems (depressive and other symptomatology) and physical problems (liver disease).

Nitrite inhalants ("poppers"---forms of amyl, butyl, and isobutyl nitrite) produce an intoxication characterized by a feeling of fullness in the head, mild euphoria, a change in the perception of time, relaxation of smooth muscles, and a possible increase in sexual feelings. In addition to the possible production of psychological dependence, these drugs carry dangers of potential impairment of immune functioning, irritation of the respiratory system, a decrease in the oxygen-carrying capacity of the blood, and a toxic reaction that can include vomiting, severe headache, hypotension, and dizziness.

Nitrous oxide ("laughing gas") causes rapid onset of an intoxication characterized by light-headedness and a floating sensation that clears in a matter of minutes after administration is stopped. There are reports of temporary but clinically relevant confusion and reversible paranoid states when nitrous oxide is used regularly.

Other substances capable of producing mild intoxications include **catnip**, which can produce states similar to those observed with marijuana and with high doses is reported to result in LSD-type perceptions; **betel nut**, which is chewed in many cultures to produce a mild euphoria and floating sensation; and **kava** (a substance derived from the South Pacific pepper plant) which produces sedation, incoordination, weight loss, mild forms of hepatitis, and lung abnormalities. In addition, individuals can develop dependence and impairment through repeated self-administration of **over-the-counter** and **prescription** drugs including **cortisol**, **antiparkisonian agents** that have cholinomimetic properties, and **antihistamines**.

304.90 Other (or Unknown) Substance Dependence (see page xx)
305.90 Other (or Unknown) Substance Abuse (see page xx)

305.90 Other (or Unknown) Substance Intoxication (see page xx)

Specify if **with perceptual disturbances:** auditory, visual, or tactile illusions; altered perceptions, or hallucinations with intact reality testing.

292.0 Other (or Unknown) Substance Withdrawal (see page xx)

Specify if **with perceptual disturbances:** auditory, visual, or tactile illusions; altered perceptions, or hallucinations with intact reality testing.

292.81 Other (or Unknown) Substance Delirium (see page xx)
292.82 Other (or Unknown) Substance Persisting Dementia (see page xx)
292.83 Other (or Unknown) Substance Persisting Amnestic Disorder (see page xx)

291.11 Other (or Unknown) Substance Psychotic Disorder, with delusions (see page xx)
291.12 Other (or Unknown) Substance Psychotic Disorder, with hallucinations (see page xx)
292.84 Other (or Unknown) Substance Mood Disorder (see page xx)
292.89 Other (or Unknown) Substance Anxiety Disorder (see page xx)
292.89 Other (or Unknown) Substance Sexual Dysfunction (see page xx)
292.89 Other (or Unknown) Substance Sleep Disorder (see page xx)
292.9 Other (or Unknown) Substance Use Disorder Not Otherwise Specified

Schizophrenia and Other Psychotic Disorders

Schizophrenia

A. Characteristic Symptoms: At least two of the following, each present for a significant portion of time during a one month period (or less if successfully treated):

    (1)   delusions
    (2)   hallucinations
    (3)   disorganized speech (e.g., frequent derailment or incoherence)
    (4)   grossly disorganized or catatonic behavior
    (5)   negative symptoms, i.e., affective flattening, alogia, or avolition

[Note: only one A symptom is required if delusions are bizarre or hallucinations consist of a voice keeping up a running commentary on the person's behavior or thoughts, or two or more voices conversing with each other].

B. Social/Occupational Dysfunction: For a significant portion of the time since the onset of the disturbance, one or more major areas of functioning such as work, interpersonal relations or self-care is markedly below the level achieved prior to the onset (or when the onset is in childhood or adolescence, failure to achieve expected level of interpersonal, academic, or occupational achievement).

C. Duration: Continuous signs of the disturbance persist for at least six months. This six-month period must include at least one month of symptoms that meet criterion A (i.e., active phase symptoms), and may include periods of prodromal or residual symptoms. During these prodromal or residual periods, the signs of the disturbance may be manifested by only negative symptoms or two or more symptoms listed in criterion A present in an attenuated form (e.g., odd beliefs, unusual perceptual experiences).

D. Schizoaffective and Mood Disorder Exclusion: Schizoaffective Disorder and Mood Disorder with Psychotic Features have been ruled out because either: (1) no major depressive or manic episodes have occurred concurrently with the active phase symptoms; or (2) if mood episodes have occurred during active phase symptoms, their total duration has been brief relative to the duration of the active and residual periods.

E. Substance/General Medical Condition Exclusion: The disturbance is not due to the direct effects of a substance (e.g., drugs of abuse, medication) or a general medical condition.

Classification of course.

- Continuous (no remission of psychotic symptoms throughout the period of observation)
- Episodic, with a progressive development of "negative" symptoms in the intervals between psychotic episodes
- Episodic, with persistent but non-progressive "negative" symptoms in the intervals between psychotic episodes
- Episodic (remittent): with complete or virtually complete remissions between psychotic episodes
- In partial remission after a single episode
- In full remission after a single episode
- Other pattern
- Period of observation less than one year

Schizophrenia Subtypes

295.30 Paranoid Type

A type of Schizophrenia in which the following criteria are met:

A. Preoccupation with one or more delusions or frequent auditory hallucinations

B. None of the following is prominent: disorganized speech, disorganized behavior, flat or inappropriate affect or catatonic behavior.

295.10 Disorganized Type

A type of Schizophrenia in which the following criteria are met:

A. All of the following are prominent:

(1) disorganized speech
(2) disorganized behavior
(3) flat or inappropriate affect

B. Does not meet criteria for Catatonic type.

295.20 Catatonic Type

A type of Schizophrenia in which the clinical picture is dominated by at least two of the following:

(1) motoric immobility as evidenced by catalepsy (including waxy flexibility) or stupor

(2) excessive motor activity (that is apparently purposeless and not influenced by external stimuli)

(3)   extreme negativism (an apparently motiveless resistance to all instructions or maintenance of a rigid posture against attempts to be moved) or mutism

(4)   peculiarities of voluntary movement as evidenced by posturing (voluntary assumption of inappropriate or bizarre postures), stereotyped movements, prominent mannerisms, or prominent grimacing

(5)   echolalia or echopraxia

295.90 Undifferentiated Type

A type of Schizophrenia in which symptoms meeting criterion A are present, but the criteria are not met for the Paranoid, Catatonic, or Disorganized types.

295.60 Residual Type

A type of Schizophrenia in which the following criteria are met:

A.   Criterion A for Schizophrenia (i.e., active phase symptoms) is no longer met, and criteria are not met for the Paranoid, Catatonic, Disorganized, and Undifferentiated types.

B.   There is continuing evidence of the disturbance, as indicated by the presence of negative symptoms or two or more symptoms listed in criterion A for Schizophrenia, present in an attenuated form (e.g., odd beliefs, unusual perceptual experiences)

295.40 Schizophreniform Disorder

A.   Meets criteria A, D, and E of Schizophrenia.

B.   An episode of the disorder (including prodromal, active, and residual phases) lasts at least one month but less than six months. (When the diagnosis must be made without waiting for recovery, it should be qualified as "provisional.")

Specify if:
Without Good Prognostic Features
With Good Prognostic Features as evidenced by at least two of the following:

(1)   onset of prominent psychotic symptoms within four weeks of the first noticeable change in usual behavior or functioning

(2)   confusion or perplexity at the height of the psychotic episode

(3)   good premorbid social and occupational functioning

I:3

(4)   absence of blunted or flat affect

295.70 Schizoaffective Disorder

A.   An uninterrupted period of illness during which, at some time, there is either a major depressive episode* or manic episode concurrent with symptoms that meet criterion A for Schizophrenia.

*Major depressive episode must include A(1) depressed mood

B.   During the same period of illness, there have been delusions or hallucinations for at least two weeks in the absence of prominent mood symptoms.

C.   Symptoms meeting criteria for a mood episode are present for a substantial portion of the total duration of the active and residual periods of the illness.

D.   Not due to the direct effects of a substance (e.g., drugs of abuse, medication) or a general medical condition.

Specify type:
    Bipolar Type: if manic episode (or both manic and major depressive episodes).
    Depressive Type: if major depressive episode only

297.1 Delusional Disorder

A.   Nonbizarre delusions (i.e., involving situations that occur in real life, such as being followed, poisoned, infected, loved at a distance, having a disease, or being deceived by one's spouse or lover) of at least one month's duration.

B.   Has never met criterion A for Schizophrenia (i.e., none of the following for more than a few hours: hallucinations, disorganized speech, grossly disorganized or catatonic behavior; or negative symptoms, i.e., affective flattening, alogia, or avolition). Note: Tactile and olfactory hallucinations are not excluded if related to the delusional theme.

C.   Apart from the impact of the delusion(s) or its ramifications, functioning is not markedly impaired and behavior is not obviously odd or bizarre.

D.   If mood episodes have occurred concurrently with delusions, their total duration has been brief relative to the duration of the delusional periods.

E.   Not due to the direct effects of a substance (e.g., drugs of abuse, medication) or a general medical condition.

I:4

Specify type: (the following types are assigned based on the predominant delusional theme)

Erotomanic Type: delusions that another person, usually of higher status, is in love with the individual.

Grandiose Type: delusions of inflated worth, power, knowledge, identity, or special relationship to a deity or famous person.

Jealous Type: delusions that one's sexual partner is unfaithful.

Persecutory Type: delusions that one (or someone to whom one is close) is being malevolently treated in some way.

Somatic Type: delusions that the person has some physical defect or general medical condition.

Mixed Type: delusions characteristic of more than one of the above types but no one theme predominates.

Unspecified Type

298.8 Brief Psychotic Disorder

A.   Presence of at least one of the following symptoms:

(1)   delusions

(2)   hallucinations

(3)   disorganized speech (e.g., frequent derailment or incoherence)

(4)   grossly disorganized or catatonic behavior

Note: do not include a symptom if it is a culturally sanctioned response pattern.

B.   Duration of an episode of the disturbance is at least one day and no more than one month, with eventual full return to premorbid level of functioning. (When the diagnosis must be made without waiting for the expected recovery, it should be qualified as "provisional.")

C.   Not better accounted for by a Mood Disorder (i.e., no full mood syndrome is present) or Schizophrenia, and not due to the direct effects of a substance (e.g., drugs of abuse, medication) or a general medical condition.

Specify if:
With Marked Stressor(s) (Brief Reactive): if symptoms occur shortly after and apparently in response to events that, singly or together, would be markedly stressful to almost anyone in similar circumstances in the person's culture.
Without Marked Stressor(s): if psychotic symptoms do <u>not</u> occur shortly after, or are not apparently in response to events that, singly or together, would be markedly stressful to almost anyone in similar circumstances in the person's culture.
With Postpartum Onset: if onset within 4 weeks postpartum.

297.3 Shared Psychotic Disorder (Folie a Deux)

A.   A delusion develops in an individual in the context of a close relationship with another person(s), who has an already established delusion.

B.   The delusion is similar in content to that of the person who already has the established delusion.

C.   Not better accounted for by another Psychotic Disorder (e.g., Schizophrenia), and not due to the direct effects of a substance (e.g., drugs of abuse, medication) or a general medical condition.

293.8x Psychotic Disorder Due to a General Medical Condition

A.   Prominent hallucinations or delusions.

B.   There is evidence from the history, physical examination, or laboratory findings of a general medical condition judged to be etiologically related to the disturbance.

C.   The disturbance does not occur exclusively during the course of Delirium or Dementia.

D.   The disturbance is not better accounted for by another mental disorder.

Code based on predominant symptom:
.x1 **With Delusions:** if delusions are the predominant symptom.
.x2 **With Hallucinations:** if hallucinations are the predominant symptom.

Substance-Induced Psychotic Disorder

A.   Prominent hallucinations or delusions. Note: Do not include hallucinations if the person has insight that they are substance-induced.

B.   There is evidence from the history, physical examination, or laboratory findings of substance intoxication or withdrawal, and the symptoms in A developed during, or within a month of, significant substance intoxication or withdrawal.

C.   The disturbance is not better accounted for by a psychotic disorder that is not substance-induced.   Evidence that the symptoms are better accounted for by a psychotic disorder that is not substance-induced might include: the symptoms precede the onset of the substance abuse or dependence; persist for a substantial period of time (e.g., about a month) after the cessation of acute withdrawal or severe intoxication; are substantially in excess of what would be expected given the character, duration, or amount of the substance used; or there is other evidence suggesting the existence of an independent non-substance-induced disorder (e.g., a history of recurrent non-substance-related episodes).

D.   The disturbance does not occur exclusively during the course of Delirium or Dementia.

Code: (Specific Substance) Psychotic Disorder
       (291.5 Alcohol, with delusions; 291.3 Alcohol, with hallucinations; 291.11 Amphetamine [or Related Substance], with delusions; 291.12 Amphetamine [or Related Substance], with hallucinations; 291.11 Cannabis, with delusions; 291.12 Cannabis, with hallucinations; 291.11 Cocaine, with delusions; 291.12 Cocaine, with hallucinations; 291.11 Hallucinogen, with delusions; 291.12 Hallucinogen, with hallucinations; 291.11 Inhalant, with delusions; 291.12 Inhalant, with hallucinations; 291.11 Opioid, with delusions; 291.12 Opioid, with hallucinations; 291.11 Phencyclidine [or Related Substance], with delusions; 291.12 Phencyclidine [or Related Substance], with hallucinations; 291.11 Sedative, Hypnotic or Anxiolytic, with delusions; 291.12 Sedative, Hypnotic or Anxiolytic, with hallucinations; 291.11 Other [or Unknown] Substance, with delusions; 291.12 Other [or Unknown] Substance, with hallucinations)

Coding note: also code substance-specific Intoxication or Withdrawal if criteria are met.

Specify if: (see table on page xx for applicability by substance)
       with onset during intoxication
       with onset during withdrawal

298.9 Psychotic Disorder Not Otherwise Specified

This category should be used to diagnose psychotic symptomatology (i.e., delusions, hallucinations, disorganized speech, grossly disorganized or catatonic behavior) about which there is inadequate information to make a specific diagnosis, or about which there is contradictory information, or for psychotic presentations that do not meet the criteria for any of the specific psychotic disorders defined above.

Examples include:

1) postpartum psychosis that does not meet criteria for Mood Disorder With Psychotic Features, Brief Psychotic Disorder, Psychotic Disorder Due to a General Medical Condition, or a Substance-Induced Psychotic Disorder.

2) persistent auditory hallucinations in the absence of any other features.

3) persistent nonbizarre delusions with periods of overlapping mood episodes that have been present for a substantial portion of the delusional disturbance.

4) psychoses with confusing clinical features that make a more specific diagnosis impossible.

5) situations in which the clinician has concluded that a psychotic disorder is present but is unable to determine whether it is primary, due to a general medical condition, or substance-induced.

Mood Disorders

Depressive Disorders

Major Depressive Episode

A. At least five of the following symptoms have been present during the same two-week period and represent a change from previous functioning; at least one of the symptoms is either (1) depressed mood or (2) loss of interest or pleasure.

   (1) depressed mood most of the day, nearly every day, as indicated by either subjective report (e.g., feels sad or empty) or observation made by others (e.g., appears tearful). Note: in children and adolescents, can be irritable mood.

   (2) markedly diminished interest or pleasure in all, or almost all, activities most of the day, nearly every day (as indicated either by subjective account or observation made by others)

   (3) significant weight loss or weight gain when not dieting (e.g., more than 5% of body weight in a month), or decrease or increase in appetite nearly every day. Note: in children, consider failure to make expected weight gains.

   (4) insomnia or hypersomnia nearly every day

   (5) psychomotor agitation or retardation nearly every day (observable by others, not merely subjective feelings of restlessness or being slowed down)

   (6) fatigue or loss of energy nearly every day

   (7) feelings of worthlessness or excessive or inappropriate guilt (which may be delusional) nearly every day (not merely self-reproach or guilt about being sick)

   (8) diminished ability to think or concentrate, or indecisiveness, nearly every day (either by subjective account or as observed by others)

   (9) recurrent thoughts of death (not just fear of dying), recurrent suicidal ideation without a specific plan, or a suicide attempt or a specific plan for committing suicide

B. The symptoms cause clinically significant distress or impairment in social, occupational, or other important areas of functioning.

C. Not due to the direct effects of a substance (e.g., drugs of abuse, medication) or a general medical condition (e.g., hypothyroidism).

D.   Not occurring within two months of the loss of a loved one (except if associated with marked functional impairment, morbid preoccupation with worthlessness, suicidal ideation, psychotic symptoms, or psychomotor retardation).

Codes For Major Depressive Episode (code in fifth digit):

.x1 - Mild: Few, if any, symptoms in excess of those required to make the diagnosis and symptoms result in only minor impairment in occupational functioning or in usual social activities or relationships with others.

.x2 - Moderate: Symptoms or functional impairment between "mild" and "severe"

.x3 - Severe without Psychotic Features: Several symptoms in excess of those required to make the diagnosis, **and** symptoms markedly interfere with occupational functioning or with usual social activities or relationships with others.

.x4 - With Psychotic Features: Delusions or hallucinations. If possible, specify whether the psychotic features are mood-congruent or mood-incongruent:

  - Mood-congruent Psychotic Features: Delusions or hallucinations whose content is entirely consistent with the typical depressive themes of personal inadequacy, guilt, disease, death, nihilism, or deserved punishment.

  - Mood-incongruent Psychotic Features: Delusions or hallucinations whose content does not involve typical depressive themes of personal inadequacy, guilt, disease, death, nihilism, or deserved punishment. Included here are such symptoms as persecutory delusions (not directly related to depressive themes), thought insertion, thought broadcasting, and delusions of control.

.x5 - In Partial Remission: Intermediate between "In Full Remission" and "Mild," **and** no previous Dysthymic Disorder. (If the Major Depressive Episode was superimposed on Dysthymic Disorder, the diagnosis of Dysthymic Disorder alone is given once the full criteria for a Major Depressive Episode are no longer met).

.x6 - In Full Remission: During the past six months no significant signs or symptoms of the disturbance.

.x0 - Unspecified

296.2x Major Depressive Disorder, Single Episode

A.   Presence of a major depressive episode (see page xx).

B.   The major depressive episode is not better accounted for by Schizoaffective Disorder, and is not superimposed on Schizophrenia, Schizophreniform Disorder, Delusional Disorder, or Psychotic Disorder NOS.

C.   Has never had a manic episode (see page xx) or unequivocal hypomanic episode (see page xx). Note: this exclusion does not apply if all of the manic or hypomanic episodes are substance- or treatment-induced

296.3x Major Depressive Disorder, Recurrent

A.   Two or more major depressive episodes (see page xx).

Note: To be considered separate episodes, there must be an interval of at least two months without significant symptoms of depression.

B.   The major depressive episodes are not due to the direct effects of a substance (e.g., drugs of abuse, medication) or a general medical condition (e.g., hypothyroidism); are not better accounted for by Schizoaffective Disorder, and are not superimposed on Schizophrenia, Schizophreniform Disorder, Delusional Disorder, or Psychotic Disorder NOS.

C.   Has never had a manic episode (see page xx) or unequivocal hypomanic episode (see page xx). Note: this exclusion does not apply if all of the manic or hypomanic episodes are substance- or treatment-induced

300.4 Dysthymic Disorder

A.   Depressed mood (or can be irritable mood in children and adolescents) for most of the day, for more days than not, as indicated either by subjective account or observation made by others, for at least two years (one year for children and adolescents).

B.   Presence, while depressed, of at least three of the following:

(1)   low self-esteem or self-confidence, or feelings of inadequacy

(2)   feelings of pessimism, despair, or hopelessness

(3)   generalized loss of interest or pleasure

(4)   social withdrawal

(5) chronic fatigue or tiredness

(6) feelings of guilt, brooding about the past

(7) subjective feelings of irritability or excessive anger

(8) decreased activity, effectiveness, or productivity

(9) difficulty in thinking reflected by poor concentration, poor memory, or indecisiveness

C. During the two year period (one-year for children or adolescents) of the disturbance, the person has never been without the symptoms in A and B for more than two months at a time.

D. No major depressive episode (see page xx) during the first two years of the disturbance (one year for children and adolescents); i.e., not better accounted for by chronic Major Depressive Disorder, or Major Depressive Disorder in partial remission.

Note: There may have been a previous major depressive episode provided there was a full remission (no significant signs or symptoms for six months) before development of the Dysthymic Disorder. In addition, after these two years (one year in children or adolescents) of Dysthymic Disorder, there may be superimposed episodes of Major Depressive Disorder in which cases both diagnoses may be given.

E. Has never had a manic episode (see page xx), or an unequivocal hypomanic episode (see page xx).

F. Does not occur exclusively during the course of a chronic psychotic disorder, such as Schizophrenia or Delusional Disorder.

G. Not due to the direct effects of a substance (e.g., drugs of abuse, medication) or a general medical condition (e.g., hypothyroidism).

Specify if:
early onset: if onset before age 21
late onset: if onset age 21 or older

311 Depressive Disorder Not Otherwise Specified

This category includes disorders with depressive features that do not meet the criteria for any specific Depressive Disorder, Adjustment Disorder With Depressed Mood, or Adjustment Disorder with Mixed Anxiety and Depressed Mood. Examples include:

1) Premenstrual dysphoric disorder: in most menstrual cycles during the past year, symptoms (e.g., markedly depressed mood, marked anxiety, marked affective lability, decreased interest in activities) regularly occurred during the last week of the luteal phase (and remitted within a few days of the onset of menses). These symptoms must be severe enough 'to markedly interfere with work, school, or usual activities. (See page xx for suggested criteria).

2) Minor depressive disorder: a disorder with episodes of two weeks of depressive symptoms but with fewer than the five items required for Major Depressive Disorder. (See page xx for suggested criteria).

3) Recurrent brief depressive disorder: a disorder with depressive episodes lasting from 2 days up to two weeks, occurring at least once a month for 12 months (not associated with the menstrual cycle). (See page xx for suggested criteria).

4) Postpsychotic depression of schizophrenia: a major depressive episode occurring during the residual phase of Schizophrenia. (See page xx for suggested criteria).

5) a major depressive episode superimposed on Delusional Disorder, Psychotic Disorder NOS, or the active phase of Schizophrenia.

6) situations in which the clinician has concluded that a depressive disorder is present but is unable to determine whether it is primary, due to a general medical condition, or substance-induced.

Bipolar Disorders

Manic Episode

A.   A distinct period of abnormally and persistently elevated, expansive, or irritable mood, lasting at least one week (or any duration if hospitalization is necessary)

B.   During the period of mood disturbance, at least three of the following symptoms have persisted (four if the mood is only irritable) and have been present to a significant degree:

(1)   inflated self-esteem or grandiosity

(2)   decreased need for sleep (e.g., feels rested after only three hours of sleep)

(3)   more talkative than usual or pressure to keep talking

(4)   flight of ideas or subjective experience that thoughts are racing

(5)   distractibility (i.e., attention too easily drawn to unimportant or irrelevant external stimuli)

(6)   increase in goal-directed activity (either socially, at work or school, or sexually) or psychomotor agitation

(7)   excessive involvement in pleasurable activities that have a high potential for painful consequences (e.g., the person engages in unrestrained buying sprees, sexual indiscretions, or foolish business investments)

C.   The mood disturbance is sufficiently severe to cause marked impairment in occupational functioning or in usual social activities or relationships with others, or to necessitate hospitalization to prevent harm to self or others

D.   Not due to the direct effects of a substance (e.g., drugs of abuse, medication) or a general medical condition (e.g., hyperthyroidism).

Note: Manic episodes that are clearly precipitated by somatic antidepressant treatment (e.g., medication, electroconvulsive therapy, light therapy) should not count towards a diagnosis of Bipolar I Disorder.

Codes for Manic Episode (code in fifth digit):

.x1 - Mild: Meets minimum symptom criteria for a manic episode.

.x2 - Moderate: Extreme increase in activity or impairment in judgment.

.x3 - Severe, without Psychotic Features: Almost continual supervision required in order to prevent physical harm to self or others.

.x4 - Severe, with Psychotic Symptoms: Delusions or hallucinations. If possible, specify whether the psychotic features are mood-congruent or mood-incongruent:

 - **Mood-congruent psychotic features:** Delusions or hallucinations whose content is entirely consistent with the typical manic themes of inflated worth, power, knowledge, identity, or special relationship to a diety or famous person.

 - **Mood-incongruent psychotic features:** Delusions or hallucinations whose content does not involve typical manic themes of inflated worth, power, knowledge, identity, or special relationship to a diety or famous person. Included are such symptoms as persecutory delusions (not directly related to grandiose ideas or themes), thought insertion, and delusions of being controlled.

.x5 - In Partial Remission: Full criteria were previously, but are not currently, met; some signs or symptoms of the disturbance have persisted.

.x6 - In Full Remission: Full criteria were previously met, but there have been no significant signs or symptoms of the disturbance for at least six months.

.x0 - Unspecified.

Hypomanic Episode

A.   A distinct period of sustained elevated, expansive, or irritable mood, lasting throughout four days, that is clearly different from the usual nondepressed mood

B.   During the period of mood disturbance, at least three of the following symptoms have persisted (four if the mood is only irritable) and have been present to a significant degree:

   (1)   inflated self-esteem or grandiosity

   (2)   decreased need for sleep (e.g., feels rested after only three hours of sleep)

   (3)   more talkative than usual or pressure to keep talking

(4)   flight of ideas or subjective experience that thoughts are racing

(5)   distractibility (i.e., attention too easily drawn to unimportant or irrelevant external stimuli)

(6)   increase in goal-directed activity (either socially, at work or school, or sexually) or psychomotor agitation

(7)   excessive involvement in pleasurable activities that have a high potential for painful consequences (e.g., the person engages in unrestrained buying sprees, sexual indiscretions, or foolish business investments)

C.   The episode is associated with an unequivocal change in functioning that is uncharacteristic of the person when not symptomatic

D.   The disturbance in mood and the change in functioning are observable by others

E.   The episode is not severe enough to cause marked impairment in social or occupational functioning, or to necessitate hospitalization, and there are no psychotic features

F.   Not due to the direct effects of a substance (e.g., drugs of abuse, medication) or a general medical condition (e.g., hyperthyroidism).

Note: Hypomanic episodes that are clearly precipitated by somatic antidepressant treatment (e.g., medication, electroconvulsive therapy, light therapy) should not count towards a diagnosis of Bipolar II Disorder.

296.0x Bipolar I Disorder, Single Manic Episode

A.   Presence of only one manic episode (see page xx) and no past major depressive episodes.

B.   The manic episode is not better accounted for by Schizoaffective Disorder, and is not superimposed on Schizophrenia, Schizophreniform Disorder, Delusional Disorder, or Psychotic Disorder NOS.

296.4x Bipolar I Disorder, Most Recent Episode Hypomanic

A.   Currently (or most recently) in a hypomanic episode (see page xx).

B.   There has previously been at least one manic episode (see page xx).

Note: To be considered separate episodes, there must be an interval of at least two months without significant symptoms of mania or hypomania, or a change in polarity.

C. The mood episodes in A and B are not better accounted for by Schizoaffective Disorder, and are not superimposed on Schizophrenia, Schizophreniform Disorder, Delusional Disorder, or Psychotic Disorder NOS.

296.4x Bipolar I Disorder, Most Recent Episode Manic

A. Currently (or most recently) in a manic episode (see page xx).

B. Either (1) or (2);

(1) there has previously been at least one major depressive episode (see page xx)

(2) there has previously been at least one hypomanic or manic episode

Note: To be considered separate episodes, there must be an interval of at least two months without significant symptoms of mania or hypomania or a change in polarity.

C. The mood episodes in A and B are not better accounted for by Schizoaffective Disorder, and are not superimposed on Schizophrenia, Schizophreniform Disorder, Delusional Disorder, or Psychotic Disorder NOS.

296.6x Bipolar I Disorder, Most Recent Episode Mixed

A. Currently (or most recently) in a mixed episode, i.e., for every day during at least a one-week period, the criteria for a major depressive episode (except for duration) and a manic episode are both met.

B. Either (1) or (2);

(1) there has previously been at least one major depressive episode (see page xx)

(2) there has previously been at least one hypomanic or manic episode

Note: To be considered separate episodes, there must be an interval of at least two months without significant symptoms of mania or hypomania or a change in polarity.

C. The mood episodes in A and B are not better accounted for by Schizoaffective Disorder, and are not superimposed on Schizophrenia, Schizophreniform Disorder, Delusional Disorder, or Psychotic Disorder NOS.

296.5x   Bipolar I Disorder, Most Recent Episode Depressed

A.   Currently (or most recently) in a major depressive episode (see page xx).

B.   There has previously been at least one manic episode (see page xx).

C.   The mood episodes in A and B are not better accounted for by Schizoaffective Disorder, and are not superimposed on Schizophrenia, Schizophreniform Disorder, Delusional Disorder, or Psychotic Disorder NOS.

296.7 Bipolar I Disorder, Most Recent Episode Unspecified

A.   Currently (or most recently) meets criteria for a manic (page xx), hypomanic (page xx) or major depressive episode (page xx) except for duration.

B.   There has previously been at least one manic episode (see page xx).

C.   The mood symptoms in A cause clinically significant distress or impairment in social, occupational, or other important areas of functioning.

D.   The mood symptoms in A and B are not better accounted for by Schizoaffective Disorder, and are not superimposed on Schizophrenia, Schizophreniform Disorder, Delusional Disorder, or Psychotic Disorder NOS.

296.89 Bipolar II Disorder (Recurrent major depressive episodes with hypomania)

A.   One or more major depressive episodes (see page xx).

B.   Presence of at least one hypomanic episode (see page xx).

Note: Hypomanic episodes that are clearly precipitated by somatic antidepressant treatment (e.g., medication, electroconvulsive therapy, light therapy) should not count toward a diagnosis of Bipolar II Disorder.

C.   Has never had a manic episode.

D.   The mood symptoms in A and B are not better accounted for by Schizoaffective Disorder, and are not superimposed on Schizophrenia, Schizophreniform Disorder, Delusional Disorder, or Psychotic Disorder NOS.

Specify Current or Most Recent Episode:
   Hypomanic: if currently (or most recently) in a hypomanic episode (see page xx)
   Depressed: if currently (or most recently) in a major depressive episode (see page xx)

301.13 Cyclothymic Disorder

A. For at least two years (one year for children and adolescents), presence of numerous periods with hypomanic symptoms (see page xx) and numerous periods with depressed mood or loss of interest or pleasure (that did not meet criteria for a major depressive episode).

B. During the above two-year period (one year in children and adolescents), the person has not been without the symptoms in A for more than two months at a time.

C. Has never met criteria for a major depressive episode (see page xx).

D. No clear evidence of a manic episode (page xx) during the first two years of the disturbance.

    Note: After the initial two years (one year in children or adolescents) of Cyclothymic Disorder, there may be superimposed manic episodes in which case both Bipolar I Disorder and Cyclothymic Disorder may be diagnosed.

E. The symptoms in A are not better accounted for by Schizoaffective Disorder, and are not superimposed on Schizophrenia, Schizophreniform Disorder, Delusional Disorder, or Psychotic Disorder NOS.

F. Not due to the direct effects of a substance (e.g., drugs of abuse, medication) or a general medical condition (e.g., hyperthyroidism).

296.80 Bipolar Disorder Not Otherwise Specified

This category includes disorders with bipolar features that do not meet criteria for any specific bipolar disorder. Examples include:

1) recurrent hypomanic episodes without intercurrent depressive symptoms

2) a manic episode superimposed on Delusional Disorder, residual Schizophrenia, or Psychotic Disorder NOS.

3) situations in which the clinician has concluded that a bipolar disorder is present but is unable to determine whether it is primary, due to a general medical condition, or substance-induced.

293.83 Mood Disorder Due to a General Medical Condition

A. A prominent and persistent disturbance in mood characterized by either (or both) of the following:

    (1) depressed mood or markedly diminished interest or pleasure in all, or almost all, activities.

    (2) elevated, expansive, or irritable mood.

B. There is evidence from the history, physical examination, or laboratory findings of a general medical condition judged to be etiologically related to the disturbance.

C. The disturbance is not better accounted for by another mental disorder (e.g., Adjustment Disorder With Depressed Mood, in response to the stress of having a general medical condition).

D. The symptoms cause clinically significant distress or impairment in social, occupational, or other important areas of functioning.

E. The disturbance does not occur exclusively during the course of Delirium or Dementia.

Specify type:
    With Manic Features: if the predominant mood is elevated, euphoric, or irritable.
    With Depressive Features: if the predominant mood is depressed.
    With Mixed Features: if symptoms of both mania and depression are present and neither predominates.

Substance-Induced Mood Disorder

A. A prominent and persistent disturbance in mood characterized by either (or both) of the following:

    (1) depressed mood or markedly diminished interest or pleasure in all, or almost all, activities

    (2) elevated, expansive, or irritable mood

B. There is evidence from the history, physical examination, or laboratory findings of substance intoxication or withdrawal, and the symptoms in A developed during, or within a month of, significant substance intoxication or withdrawal.

C. The disturbance is not better accounted for by a Mood Disorder that is not substance-induced. Evidence that the symptoms are better accounted for by a Mood Disorder that is not substance-induced might include: the symptoms precede the onset of the substance abuse or dependence; persist for a substantial period of time (e.g., about a month) after the cessation of acute withdrawal or severe intoxication; are substantially in excess of what would be expected given the character, duration, or amount of the substance used; or there is other evidence suggesting the existence of an independent non-substance-induced mood disorder (e.g., a history of recurrent non-substance-related major depressive episodes).

D. The symptoms cause clinically significant distress or impairment in social, occupational, or other important areas of functioning.

E. The disturbance does not occur exclusively during the course of Delirium.

Code: (Specific Substance) Mood Disorder
(291.8 Alcohol, 292.84 Amphetamine [or Related Substance], 292.84 Cocaine, 292.84 Hallucinogen, 292.84 Inhalant, 292.84 Opioid, 292.84 Phencyclidine [or Related Substance], 292.84 Sedative, Hypnotic, or Anxiolytic, 292.84 Other [or Unknown] Substance)

Coding note: also code substance-specific Intoxication or Withdrawal if criteria are met.

Specify type:
With Manic Features: if the predominant mood is elevated, euphoric, or irritable.
With Depressive Features: if the predominant mood is depressed.
With Mixed Features: if symptoms of both mania and depression are present and neither predominates.

Specify if: (see table on page xx for applicability by substance)
with onset during intoxication
with onset during withdrawal

296.90 Mood Disorder Not Otherwise Specified

This category includes disorders with mood symptoms that do not meet the criteria for any specific mood disorder and in which it is difficult to choose between Depressive Disorder NOS and Bipolar Disorder NOS (e.g., acute agitation).

Cross-Sectional Symptom Features

Specify if: **With Melancholic Features** (can be applied to major depressive episodes occurring in Major Depressive Disorder, Bipolar I Disorder or Bipolar II Disorder):

A.   Either of the following, occurring during the most severe period of the current episode:

(1)   Loss of pleasure in all, or almost all, activities.

(2)   Lack of reactivity to usually pleasurable stimuli (does not feel much better, even temporarily, when something good happens).

B.   At least three of the following:

(1)   distinct quality of depressed mood (i.e., the depressed mood is perceived as distinctly different from the kind of feeling experienced after the death of a loved one)

(2)   the depression is regularly worse in the morning

(3)   early morning awakening (at least two hours before usual time of awakening)

(4)   marked psychomotor retardation or agitation

(5)   significant anorexia or weight loss

(6)   excessive or inappropriate guilt

Specify if: **With Atypical Features** (can be applied to the most recent major depressive episode in Major Depressive Disorder, Bipolar I Disorder, or Bipolar II Disorder, or to Dysthymic Disorder):

A. Mood reactivity (i.e., mood brightens in response to actual or potential positive events).

B. Two of the following features, present for most of the time, for at least two weeks:

  (1) significant weight gain or increase in appetite

  (2) hypersomnia

  (3) leaden paralysis (i.e., heavy, leaden feelings in arms or legs)

  (4) long-standing pattern of interpersonal rejection sensitivity (not limited to episodes of mood disturbance) resulting in significant social or occupational impairment

C. Does not meet criteria for "With Melancholic Features" during the same episode.

Specify if: **With Catatonic Features** (can be applied to the most recent manic episode or major depressive episode in Major Depressive Disorder, Bipolar I Disorder, or Bipolar II Disorder):

The clinical picture is dominated by at least two of the following:

  (1) motoric immobility as evidenced by catalepsy (including waxy flexibility) or stupor

  (2) excessive motor activity (that is apparently purposeless and not influenced by external stimuli)

  (3) extreme negativism (an apparently motiveless resistance to all instructions or maintenance of a rigid posture against attempts to be moved) or mutism

  (4) peculiarities of voluntary movement as evidenced by posturing (voluntary assumption of inappropriate or bizarre postures), stereotyped movements, prominent mannerisms, or prominent grimacing

  (5) echolalia or echopraxia

Course Specifiers:

Specify if: **With Rapid Cycling** (can be applied to Bipolar I Disorder or Bipolar II Disorder):

At least four episodes of a mood disturbance in the previous 12 months that meet criteria for a manic episode, a hypomanic episode, or a major depressive episode.

Note: episodes are demarcated by a switch to an episode of opposite polarity (e.g., depressed mood to manic mood) or by a period of remission.

Specify if: **With Seasonal Pattern** (can be applied to Bipolar I Disorder, Bipolar II Disorder, and Major Depressive Disorder, Recurrent):

A. There has been a regular temporal relationship between the onset of an episode of Bipolar I or Bipolar II Disorder or Major Depressive Disorder, Recurrent, and a particular time of the year (e.g., regular appearance of depression in the fall or winter).

B. Full remissions (or a change from depression to mania or hypomania) also occur at a characteristic time of the year (e.g., depression disappears in the spring).

C. In the last two years, two episodes have occurred that demonstrate the temporal seasonal relationship defined in A and B, and no nonseasonal episodes have occurred during that same period.

D. Seasonal episodes of mood disturbance, as described above, substantially outnumber any nonseasonal episodes of such disturbance that may have occurred over the individual's lifetime.

Specify if: **With Postpartum Onset** (can be applied to major depressive or manic episodes in Bipolar I Disorder, Bipolar II Disorder, or Major Depressive Disorder; or to Brief Psychotic Disorder):

Onset of episode within 4 weeks postpartum.

Longitudinal Course Specifiers for Major Depressive Disorder:

Specify: **With Full Interepisode Recovery**, if no prominent mood symptoms between two most recent major depressive episodes.
Without Full Interepisode Recovery, if prominent mood symptoms between two most recent major depressive episodes.

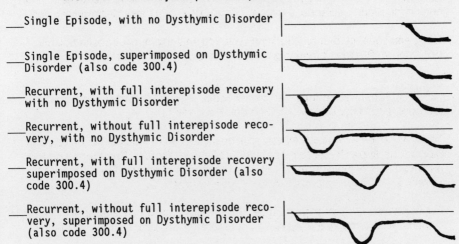

___Single Episode, with no Dysthymic Disorder

___Single Episode, superimposed on Dysthymic Disorder (also code 300.4)

___Recurrent, with full interepisode recovery with no Dysthymic Disorder

___Recurrent, without full interepisode recovery, with no Dysthymic Disorder

___Recurrent, with full interepisode recovery superimposed on Dysthymic Disorder (also code 300.4)

___Recurrent, without full interepisode recovery, superimposed on Dysthymic Disorder (also code 300.4)

Longitudinal Course Specifiers for Bipolar I Disorder:

Specify: **With Full Interepisode Recovery**, if no prominent mood symptoms between two most recent manic or major depressive episodes.
Without Full Interepisode Recovery, if prominent mood symptoms between two most recent manic or major depressive episodes.

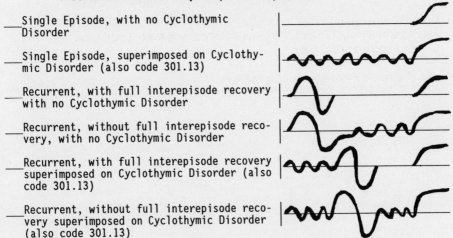

___Single Episode, with no Cyclothymic Disorder

___Single Episode, superimposed on Cyclothymic Disorder (also code 301.13)

___Recurrent, with full interepisode recovery with no Cyclothymic Disorder

___Recurrent, without full interepisode recovery, with no Cyclothymic Disorder

___Recurrent, with full interepisode recovery superimposed on Cyclothymic Disorder (also code 301.13)

___Recurrent, without full interepisode recovery superimposed on Cyclothymic Disorder (also code 301.13)

Anxiety Disorders

Panic Attack

A discrete period of intense fear or discomfort, in which at least four of the following symptoms developed abruptly and reached a peak within 10 minutes:

(1) palpitations, pounding heart, or accelerated heart rate

(2) sweating

(3) trembling or shaking

(4) sensations of shortness of breath or smothering

(5) feeling of choking

(6) chest pain or discomfort

(7) nausea or abdominal distress

(8) feeling dizzy, unsteady, lightheaded, or faint

(9) derealization (feelings of unreality) or depersonalization (being detached from oneself)

(10) fear of losing control or going crazy

(11) fear of dying

(12) paresthesias (numbness or tingling sensations)

(13) chills or hot flushes

Panic attacks can occur in a variety of Anxiety Disorders (e.g., Panic Disorder, Social Phobia, Simple Phobia, Posttraumatic Stress Disorder). In determining the differential diagnostic significance of a panic attack, it is important to consider the context in which the panic attack occurs. There are two prototypical relationships between the onset of a panic attack and situational triggers: 1) **unexpected (uncued)** panic attacks, in which the onset of the panic attack is not associated with a situational trigger (i.e., occurring "out of the blue"); and 2) **situationally bound (cued)** panic attacks, in which a panic attack almost invariably occurs immediately upon exposure to, or in anticipation of, the situational trigger ("cue"). The occurrence of unexpected panic attacks is required for a diagnosis of Panic Disorder, while situationally bound panic attacks are most characteristic of Social and Specific Phobias.

Moreover, there are panic attack presentations that do not conform to either of these prototypical relationships. These **situationally predisposed** panic attacks are more likely to occur upon exposure to the situational trigger ("cue") but are not invariably associated with the cue. In addition, these panic attacks may not necessarily occur immediately after the exposure. There is some evidence that situationally predisposed panic attacks are especially frequent in Panic Disorder but may at times occur in Specific Phobia or Social Phobia.

The differential diagnosis of panic attacks is complicated by the fact that an exclusive relationship does not exist between the type of panic attack and the diagnosis. For instance, although Panic Disorder definitionally requires that at least some of the panic attacks be unexpected, individuals with a disturbance meeting the criteria for this disorder frequently have attacks that are cued, particularly later in the course of the disorder.

There are limitations in how specific the criteria sets can be in defining the boundaries between disorders in this section, since they must necessarily emphasize the prototypic presentations of each disorder. The diagnostic issues for difficult boundary cases will be discussed in the differential diagnosis section of the text for each of these disorders.

Panic Disorder

300.01 Panic Disorder Without Agoraphobia

A. Both (1) and (2):

   (1) recurrent unexpected panic attacks

   (2) at least one of the attacks has been followed by a month (or more) of: (a) persistent concern about having additional attacks; (b) worry about the implications of the attack or its consequences (e.g., losing control, having a heart attack, "going crazy"); or (c) a significant change in behavior related to the attacks

B. Absence of Agoraphobia (defined below).

C. The panic attacks are not due to the direct effects of a substance (e.g., drugs of abuse, medication) or a general medical condition (e.g., hyperthyroidism).

D. The anxiety is not better accounted for by another mental disorder, such as Obsessive-Compulsive Disorder (e.g., fear of contamination), Posttraumatic Stress Disorder (e.g., in response to stimuli associated with a severe stressor), Separation Anxiety Disorder, or Social Phobia (e.g., fear of embarrassment in social situations).

300.21 Panic Disorder With Agoraphobia

A.   Both (1) and (2):

   (1)   recurrent unexpected panic attacks

   (2)   at least one of the attacks has been followed by a month (or more) of: (a) persistent concern about having additional attacks; (b) worry about the implications of the attack or its consequences (e.g., losing control, having a heart attack, "going crazy"); or (c) a significant change in behavior related to the attacks

B.   The presence of agoraphobia, i.e., anxiety about being in places or situations from which escape might be difficult (or embarrassing) or in which help may not be available in the event of having an unexpected or situationally predisposed panic attack. Agoraphobic fears typically involve characteristic clusters of situations that include being outside the home alone; being in a crowd or standing in a line; being on a bridge; and traveling in a bus, train, or car.

   Note: Consider the diagnosis of Specific Phobia if limited to one or only a few specific situations, or Social Phobia if the avoidance is limited to social situations.

C.   Agoraphobic situations are avoided (e.g., travel is restricted), or else endured with marked distress or with anxiety about having a panic attack, or require the presence of a companion.

D.   The panic attacks are not due to the direct effects of a substance (e.g., drugs of abuse, medication) or a general medical condition (e.g., hyperthyroidism).

E.   The anxiety or phobic avoidance is not better accounted for by another mental disorder, such as Specific Phobia (e.g., avoidance limited to a single situation like elevators), Separation Anxiety Disorder (e.g., avoidance of school), Obsessive-Compulsive Disorder (e.g., fear of contamination), Posttraumatic Stress Disorder (e.g., avoidance of stimuli associated with a severe stressor), or Social Phobia (e.g., avoidance limited to social situations because of fear of embarrassment).

300.22 Agoraphobia Without History of Panic Disorder

A. The presence of agoraphobia, i.e., anxiety about being in places or situations from which escape might be difficult (or embarrassing) or in which help may not be available in the event of suddenly developing panic-like symptoms that the individual fears could be incapacitating or extremely embarrassing, for example, fear of going outside because of fear of having a sudden episode of dizziness or a sudden attack of diarrhea. Agoraphobic fears typically involve characteristic clusters of situations that include being outside the home alone; being in a crowd or standing in a line; being on a bridge; and traveling in a bus, train, or car.

B. Agoraphobic situations are avoided (e.g., travel is restricted), or else endured with marked distress or with anxiety about having panic-like symptoms, or require the presence of a companion.

C. Has never met criteria for Panic Disorder.

D. If an associated general medical condition is present, the fear described in criterion A is clearly in excess of that usually associated with the condition.

E. The anxiety or phobic avoidance is not better accounted for by another mental disorder, such as Specific Phobia (e.g., avoidance limited to a single situation like elevators), Separation Anxiety Disorder (e.g., avoidance of school), Obsessive-Compulsive Disorder (e.g., fear of contamination), Posttraumatic Stress Disorder (e.g., avoidance of stimuli associated with a severe stressor), or Social Phobia (e.g., avoidance limited to social situations because of fear of embarrassment).

F. Not due to the direct effects of a substance (e.g., drugs of abuse, medication) or a general medical condition.

300.29 Specific Phobia

A. Marked and persistent fear that is excessive or unreasonable, cued by the presence or anticipation of a specific object or situation (e.g., flying, heights, animals, receiving an injection, seeing blood).

B. Exposure to the phobic stimulus almost invariably provokes an immediate anxiety response, which may take the form of a situationally bound or situationally predisposed panic attack. Note: in children, the anxiety may be expressed by crying, tantrums, freezing, or clinging.

C. The person recognizes that the fear is excessive or unreasonable. Note: in children, this feature may be absent.

D. The phobic situation(s) is avoided, or else endured with intense anxiety or distress.

E. The avoidance, anxious anticipation, or distress in the feared situations interferes significantly with the person's normal routine, occupational (academic) functioning, or with social activities or relationships with others, or there is marked distress about having the phobia.

F. The anxiety, panic attacks, or phobic avoidance associated with the specific object or situation are not better accounted for by another mental disorder, such as Obsessive-Compulsive Disorder (e.g., fear of contamination), Posttraumatic Stress Disorder (e.g., avoidance of stimuli associated with a severe stressor), Separation Anxiety Disorder (e.g., avoidance of school), Social Phobia (e.g., avoidance of social situations because of fear of embarrassment), Panic Disorder with Agoraphobia, or Agoraphobia Without History of Panic Disorder.

Specify type:
Animal Type
Natural Environment Type (e.g., heights, storms, and water)
Blood, Injection, Injury Type
Situational Type (e.g., planes, elevators, or enclosed places)
Other Type (e.g., phobic avoidance of situations that may lead to choking, vomiting, or contracting an illness; or in children, avoidance of loud sounds or costumed characters)

300.23 Social Phobia (Social Anxiety Disorder)

A. A marked and persistent fear of one or more social or performance situations in which the person is exposed to unfamiliar people or to possible scrutiny by others. The individual fears that he or she will act in a way (or show anxiety symptoms) that will be humiliating or embarrassing. Note: in children, there must be evidence of capacity for social relationships with familiar people and the anxiety must occur in peer settings, not just in interactions with adults.

B. Exposure to the feared social situation almost invariably provokes anxiety, which may take the form of a situationally bound or situationally predisposed panic attack. Note: In children, the anxiety may be expressed by crying, tantrums, freezing, or withdrawal from the social situation.

C. The person recognizes that the fear is excessive or unreasonable. Note: in children, this feature may be absent.

D. The feared social or performance situations are avoided, or else endured with intense anxiety or distress.

E.   The avoidance, anxious anticipation, or distress in the feared social or performance situation(s) interferes significantly with the person's normal routine, occupational (academic) functioning, or with social activities or relationships with others, or there is marked distress about having the phobia.

F.   The fear or avoidance is not due to the direct effects of a substance (e.g., drugs of abuse, medication) or a general medical condition, and is not better accounted for by Panic Disorder With or Without Agoraphobia, Separation Anxiety Disorder, Body Dysmorphic Disorder, a Pervasive Developmental Disorder, or Schizoid Personality Disorder.

G.   If a general medical condition or other mental disorder is present, the fear in A is unrelated to it, e.g., the fear is not of stuttering, trembling (in Parkinson's disease) or exhibiting abnormal eating behavior (in Anorexia Nervosa or Bulimia Nervosa).

Specify if **Generalized Type:** if the fears include most social situations (also consider the additional diagnosis of Avoidant Personality Disorder).

300.3 Obsessive-Compulsive Disorder

A.   Either obsessions or compulsions:

Obsessions as defined by (1), (2), (3), and (4):

(1)   recurrent and persistent thoughts, impulses, or images that are experienced, at some time during the disturbance, as intrusive and inappropriate, and cause marked anxiety or distress

(2)   the thoughts, impulses, or images are not simply excessive worries about real-life problems

(3)   the person attempts to ignore or suppress such thoughts or impulses or to neutralize them with some other thought or action

(4)   the person recognizes that the obsessional thoughts, impulses, or images are a product of his or her own mind (not imposed from without as in thought insertion)

Compulsions as defined by (1) and (2):

   (1)   repetitive behaviors (e.g., handwashing, ordering, checking) or mental acts
         (e.g., praying, counting, repeating words silently) that the person feels driven to
         perform in response to an obsession, or according to rules that must be applied
         rigidly

   (2)   the behaviors or mental acts are aimed at preventing or reducing distress or
         preventing some dreaded event or situation; however these behaviors or mental
         acts either are not connected in a realistic way with what they are designed to
         neutralize or prevent, or are clearly excessive

B.   At some point during the course of the disorder, the person has recognized that
     the obsessions or compulsions are excessive or unreasonable. Note: this does
     not apply to children.

C.   The obsessions or compulsions cause marked distress; are time-consuming (take
     more than an hour a day); or significantly interfere with the person's normal routine,
     occupational functioning, or usual social activities or relationships with others.

D.   If another Axis I disorder is present, the content of the obsessions or compulsions
     is not restricted to it (e.g., preoccupation with food in the presence of an Eating
     Disorder; hair pulling in the presence of Trichotillomania; concern with appearance
     in the presence of Body Dysmorphic Disorder; preoccupation with drugs in the
     presence of a Substance Use Disorder; preoccupation with having a serious illness
     in the presence of Hypochondriasis; or guilty ruminations in the presence of Major
     Depressive Disorder).

E.   Not due to the direct effects of a substance (e.g., drugs of abuse, medication) or a
     general medical condition.

   Specify if **Poor Insight Type:** if, for most of the time during the current episode, the
         person does not recognize that the obsessions and compulsions are excessive
         or unreasonable

309.81 Posttraumatic Stress Disorder

A.   The person has been exposed to a traumatic event in which both of the following have been present:

    (1)   the person has experienced, witnessed, or been confronted with an event or events that involve actual or threatened death or serious injury, or a threat to the physical integrity of oneself or others

    (2)   the person's response involved intense fear, helplessness, or horror. Note: in children, it may be expressed instead by disorganized or agitated behavior

B.   The traumatic event is persistently reexperienced in at least one of the following ways:

    (1)   recurrent and intrusive distressing recollections of the event, including images, thoughts, or perceptions. Note: in young children, repetitive play may occur in which themes or aspects of the trauma are expressed

    (2)   recurrent distressing dreams of the event. Note: in children, there may be frightening dreams without recognizable content

    (3)   acting or feeling as if the traumatic event were recurring (includes a sense of reliving the experience, illusions, hallucinations, and dissociative flashback episodes, including those that occur upon awakening or when intoxicated) Note: in young children, trauma-specific reenactment may occur.

    (4)   intense psychological distress at exposure to internal or external cues that symbolize or resemble an aspect of the traumatic event

    (5)   physiologic reactivity upon exposure to internal or external cues that symbolize or resemble an aspect of the traumatic event

C.   Persistent avoidance of stimuli associated with the trauma and numbing of general responsiveness (not present before the trauma), as indicated by at least three of the following:

    (1) efforts to avoid thoughts, feelings, or conversations associated with the trauma

    (2) efforts to avoid activities, places, or people that arouse recollections of the trauma

    (3) inability to recall an important aspect of the trauma

    (4) markedly diminished interest or participation in significant activities

    (5) feeling of detachment or estrangement from others

(6) restricted range of affect (e.g., unable to have loving feelings)

(7) sense of a foreshortened future (e.g., does not expect to have a career, marriage, children, or a normal life span)

D. Persistent symptoms of increased arousal (not present before the trauma), as indicated by at least two of the following:

(1) difficulty falling or staying asleep

(2) irritability or outbursts of anger

(3) difficulty concentrating

(4) hypervigilance

(5) exaggerated startle response

E. Duration of the disturbance (symptoms in B, C, and D) is more than one month.

F. The disturbance causes clinically significant distress or impairment in social, occupational, or other important areas of functioning.

Specify if:
Acute: if duration of symptoms is less than three months
Chronic: if duration of symptoms is three months or more

Specify if:
With Delayed Onset: onset of symptoms at least six months after the stressor

308.3 Acute Stress Disorder

A. The person has been exposed to a traumatic event in which both of the following have been present:

(1) the person has experienced, witnessed, or been confronted with an event or events that involve actual or threatened death or serious injury, or a threat to the physical integrity of oneself or others.

(2) the person's response involved intense fear, helplessness, or horror

B.   Either while experiencing, or immediately after experiencing, the distressing event, the individual has at least three of the following dissociative symptoms:

    (1)   subjective sense of numbing, detachment, or absence of emotional responsiveness

    (2)   a reduction in awareness of one's surroundings (e.g., "being in a daze")

    (3)   derealization

    (4)   depersonalization

    (5)   dissociative amnesia, i.e., inability to recall an important aspect of the trauma

C.   The traumatic event is persistently reexperienced in at least one of the following ways: recurrent images, thoughts, dreams, illusions, flashback episodes, or a sense of reliving the experience; or distress upon exposure to reminders of the traumatic event.

D.   Marked avoidance of stimuli that arouse recollections of the trauma (e.g., thoughts, feelings, conversations, activities, places or people)

E.   Marked symptoms of anxiety or increased arousal (e.g., difficulty sleeping, irritability, poor concentration, hypervigilance, exaggerated startle response, and motor restlessness)

F.   The disturbance causes clinically significant distress or impairment in social, occupational, or other important areas of functioning, or the individual is prevented from pursuing some necessary task, such as obtaining necessary medical or legal assistance or mobilizing personal resources by telling family members about the traumatic experience

G.   The symptoms last for a minimum of two days and a maximum of four weeks and occur within four weeks of the traumatic event.

H.   Not due to the direct effects of a substance (e.g., drugs of abuse, medication) or a general medical condition, and is not merely an exacerbation of a preexisting Axis I or Axis II disorder.

300.02 Generalized Anxiety Disorder (includes Overanxious Disorder of Childhood)

A.   Excessive anxiety and worry (apprehensive expectation), occurring more days than not for at least six months, about a number of events or activities (such as work or school performance)

B.   The person finds it difficult to control the worry.

C.   The anxiety and worry are associated with at least three of the following six symptoms (with at least some symptoms present for more days than not for the past six months):

   (1)   restlessness or feeling keyed up or on edge

   (2)   being easily fatigued

   (3)   difficulty concentrating or mind going blank

   (4)   irritability

   (5)   muscle tension

   (6)   sleep disturbance (difficulty falling or staying asleep, or restless unsatisfying sleep)

D.   The focus of the anxiety and worry is not confined to features of an Axis I disorder, e.g., the anxiety or worry is not about having a panic attack (as in Panic Disorder), being embarrassed in public (as in Social Phobia), being contaminated (as in Obsessive-Compulsive Disorder), being away from home or close relatives (as in Separation Anxiety Disorder), gaining weight (as in Anorexia Nervosa), or having a serious illness (as in Hypochondriasis), and is not part of Posttraumatic Stress Disorder.

E.   The anxiety, worry, or physical symptoms cause clinically significant distress or impairment in social, occupational, or other important areas of functioning.

F.   Not due to the direct effects of a substance (e.g., drugs of abuse, medication) or a general medical condition (e.g., hyperthyroidism), and does not occur exclusively during a Mood Disorder, Psychotic Disorder, or a Pervasive Developmental Disorder.

293.89 Anxiety Disorder Due to a General Medical Condition

A. Prominent anxiety, panic attacks, obsessions or compulsions.

B. There is evidence from the history, physical examination, or laboratory findings of a general medical condition judged to be etiologically related to the disturbance.

C. The disturbance is not better accounted for by another mental disorder (e.g., Adjustment Disorder With Anxiety, in which the stressor is a serious medical illness).

D. The disturbance causes clinically significant distress or impairment in social, occupational, or other important areas of functioning.

E. The disturbance does not occur exclusively during the course of Delirium or Dementia.

Specify if:
With Generalized Anxiety
With Panic Attacks
With Obsessive-Compulsive symptoms

Substance-Induced Anxiety Disorder

A. Prominent anxiety, panic attacks, obsessions or compulsions.

B. There is evidence from the history, physical examination, or laboratory findings of substance intoxication or withdrawal, and the symptoms in A developed during, or within a month of, significant substance intoxication or withdrawal.

C. The disturbance is not better accounted for by an Anxiety Disorder that is not substance-induced. Evidence that the symptoms are better accounted for by an Anxiety Disorder that is not substance-induced might include: the symptoms precede the onset of the substance abuse or dependence; persist for a substantial period of time (e.g., about a month) after the cessation of acute withdrawal or severe intoxication; are substantially in excess of what would be expected given the character, duration, or amount of the substance used; or there is other evidence suggesting the existence of an independent non-substance-induced Anxiety Disorder (e.g., a history of recurrent non-substance-related panic attacks).

D. The disturbance causes clinically significant distress or impairment in social, occupational, or other important areas of functioning.

E. The disturbance does not occur exclusively during the course of Delirium or Dementia.

Code: (Specific Substance) Anxiety Disorder
(291.8 Alcohol, 292.84 Amphetamine (or Related Substance), 292.84 Caffeine, 292.84 Cannabis, 292.84 Cocaine, 292.84 Hallucinogen, 292.84 Inhalant, 292.84 Phencyclidine (or Related Substance), 292.84 Sedative, Hypnotic, or Anxiolytic, 292.84 Other [or Unknown] Substance)

Coding note: also code substance-specific Intoxication or Withdrawal if criteria are met.

Specify if:
With Generalized Anxiety
With Panic Attacks
With Obsessive-Compulsive Symptoms

Specify if: (see table on page xx for applicability by substance)
with onset during intoxication
with onset during withdrawal

300.00 Anxiety Disorder Not Otherwise Specified

This category includes disorders with prominent anxiety or phobic avoidance that do not meet criteria for any specific Anxiety Disorder, Adjustment Disorder with Anxiety, or Adjustment Disorder with Mixed Anxiety and Depressed Mood. Examples include:

1) Mixed anxiety-depressive disorder: clinically significant symptoms of anxiety and depression but the criteria are not met for either a specific Mood or Anxiety Disorder (see page xx for suggested criteria).

2) fear that one's physical appearance or body odor is offensive to other individuals, leading to social avoidance.

3) clinically significant social phobic symptoms related to the social impact of having a general medical condition or mental disorder (e.g., Parkinson's disease, dermatologic conditions, Stuttering, Anorexia Nervosa).

4) situations in which the clinician has concluded that an Anxiety Disorder is present but is unable to determine whether it is primary, due to a general medical condition, or substance-induced.

Somatoform Disorders

300.81 Somatization Disorder

A.   A history of many physical complaints beginning before the age of 30, occurring over a period of several years, and resulting in treatment being sought or significant impairment in social or occupational functioning.

B.   Each of the following criteria must have been met at some time during the course of the disorder. To count a symptom as significant, it must not be fully explained by a known general medical condition, or the resulting complaints or impairment are in excess of what would be expected from the history, physical examination, or laboratory findings.

   (1)   Four pain symptoms: A history of pain related to at least four different sites or functions (such as head, abdomen, back, joints, extremities, chest, rectum, during sexual intercourse, during menstruation, or during urination)

   (2)   Two gastrointestinal symptoms: A history of at least two gastrointestinal symptoms other than pain (such as nausea, diarrhea, bloating, vomiting other than during pregnancy, or intolerance of several different foods)

   (3)   One sexual symptom: A history of at least one sexual or reproductive symptom other than pain (such as sexual indifference, erectile or ejaculatory dysfunction, irregular menses, excessive menstrual bleeding, vomiting throughout pregnancy)

   (4)   One pseudoneurologic symptom: A history of at least one symptom or deficit suggesting a neurological disorder not limited to pain (conversion symptoms such as blindness, double vision, deafness, loss of touch or pain sensation, hallucinations, aphonia, impaired coordination or balance, paralysis or localized weakness, difficulty swallowing, difficulty breathing, urinary retention, seizures; dissociative symptoms such as amnesia, or loss of consciousness other than fainting)

300.11 Conversion Disorder

A.   One or more symptoms or deficits affecting voluntary motor or sensory function suggesting a neurological or general medical condition.

B.   Psychological factors are judged to be associated with the symptom or deficit because the initiation or exacerbation of the symptom or deficit is preceded by conflicts or other stressors.

C.   The symptom or deficit is not intentionally produced or feigned (as in Factitious Disorder or Malingering).

D.   The symptom or deficit cannot, after appropriate investigation, be fully explained by a neurological or general medical condition, and is not a culturally sanctioned behavior or experience.

E.   The symptom or deficit causes clinically significant distress or impairment in social, occupational, or other important areas of functioning; or warrants medical evaluation.

F.   The symptom or deficit is not limited to pain or sexual dysfunction, does not occur exclusively during the course of Somatization Disorder, and is not better accounted for by another mental disorder.

Specify type of symptom or deficit:
 With Motor Symptom or Deficit
 With Seizures or Convulsions
 With Sensory Symptom or Deficit
 With Mixed Presentation

300.7 Hypochondriasis

A.   Preoccupation with fears of having, or the idea that one has, a serious disease based on the person's misinterpretation of bodily symptoms.

B.   The preoccupation persists despite appropriate medical evaluation and reassurance.

C.   The belief in A is not of delusional intensity (as in Delusional Disorder, Somatic Type) and is not restricted to a circumscribed concern about appearance (as in Body Dysmorphic Disorder).

D.   The preoccupation causes clinically significant distress or impairment in social, occupational, or other important areas of functioning.

E.   The duration of the disturbance is at least six months.

F.   The preoccupation does not occur exclusively during the course of Generalized Anxiety Disorder, Obsessive-Compulsive Disorder, Panic Disorder, a major depressive episode, Separation Anxiety, or another Somatoform Disorder.

Specify if: **with poor insight:** if, for most of the time during the current episode, the person does not recognize that the concern about having a serious illness is excessive or unreasonable

300.71 Body Dysmorphic Disorder

A. Preoccupation with an imagined defect in appearance. If a slight physical anomaly is present, the person's concern is markedly excessive.

B. The preoccupation causes clinically significant distress or impairment in social, occupational, or other important areas of functioning.

C. The preoccupation is not better accounted for by another mental disorder (e.g., dissatisfaction with body shape and size in Anorexia Nervosa).

Pain Disorder

A. Pain in one or more anatomical sites is the predominant focus of the clinical presentation and is of sufficient severity to warrant clinical attention.

B. The pain causes clinically significant distress or impairment in social, occupational, or other important areas of functioning.

C. Psychological factors are judged to have an important role in the onset, severity, exacerbation, or maintenance of the pain.

D. The pain is not better accounted for by a Mood, Anxiety, or Psychotic Disorder and does not meet criteria for Dyspareunia.

Code as follows:

307.80 Pain Disorder Associated with Psychological Factors: psychological factors are judged to have a major role in the onset, severity, exacerbation, or maintenance of the pain. (If a general medical condition is present, it does not have a major role in the onset, severity, exacerbation, or maintenance of the pain). Do not diagnose if criteria are also met for Somatization Disorder.

307.89 Pain Disorder Associated with Both Psychological Factors and a General Medical Condition: both psychological factors and a general medical condition are judged to have important roles in the onset, severity, exacerbation, or maintenance of the pain.

Specify if:
> **Acute** (duration of less than six months)
> **Chronic** (duration of six months or more)

Note: the following is included here to facilitate differential diagnosis and should be coded on Axis III.

> **Pain Disorder Associated with a General Medical Condition:** a general medical condition has a major role in the onset, severity, exacerbation, or maintenance of the pain. (If psychological factors are present, they are not judged to have a major role in the onset, severity, exacerbation, or maintenance of the pain).

Code on Axis III based on anatomic site: abdominal (789.0), back (724.5), breast (611.71), chest (786.50), ear (388.70), eye (379.91), headache (784.0), joint (719.40), limb (729.5), pelvic (625.9), renal colic (788.0), shoulder (719.41), throat (784.1), tongue (529.6), tooth (525.9), urinary (788.0).

300.82 Undifferentiated Somatoform Disorder

A.   One or more physical complaints (e.g., fatigue, loss of appetite, gastrointestinal or urinary complaints)

B.   Either (1) or (2);

   (1)   after appropriate investigation, the symptoms cannot be explained by a known general medical condition or pathophysiologic mechanism (e.g., the effects of injury, medication, drugs, or alcohol)

   (2)   when there is a related general medical condition, the physical complaints or resulting social or occupational impairment are grossly in excess of what would be expected from the physical findings

C.   The symptoms cause clinically significant distress or impairment in social, occupational, or other important areas of functioning.

D.   The duration of the disturbance is at least six months

E.   Does not occur exclusively during the course of another mental disorder (e.g., another Somatoform Disorder, Sexual Dysfunction, Mood Disorder, Anxiety Disorder, Sleep Disorder, or Psychotic Disorder).

300.89 Somatoform Disorder Not Otherwise Specified

This category is for disorders with somatoform symptoms that do not meet the criteria for any specific Somatoform Disorder. Examples include:

1) Pseudocyesis: a false belief of being pregnant associated with objective signs of pregnancy, which may include abdominal enlargement (although the umbilicus does not become everted), reduced menstrual flow, amenorrhea, subjective sensation of fetal movement, nausea, breast engorgement and secretions, and labor pains at the expected date of delivery. Endocrine changes may be present but the syndrome cannot be explained by a general medical condition causing endocrine changes (e.g., hormone-secreting tumor).

2) complaints of fatigue or body weakness not due to another mental disorder of less than six months' duration.

3) a disorder involving nonpsychotic hypochondriacal symptoms of less than six months' duration.

4) a disorder involving physical complaints of less than six months' duration.

Factitious Disorders

Factitious Disorder

A.   Intentional production or feigning of physical or psychological signs or symptoms.

B.   The motivation for the behavior is to assume the sick role.

C.   External incentives for the behavior (such as economic gain, avoiding legal responsibility, or improving physical well-being, as in Malingering) are absent.

D.   The behavior is not better accounted for by another mental disorder.

Code based on type:

300.16 With Predominantly Psychological Signs and Symptoms: if psychological signs and symptoms predominate in the clinical presentation.

300.17 With Predominantly Physical Signs and Symptoms: if physical signs and symptoms predominate in the clinical presentation.

300.18 With Combined Psychological and Physical Signs and Symptoms: if both psychological and physical signs and symptoms are present but neither predominate in the clinical presentation.

300.19 Factitious Disorder Not Otherwise Specified

This category is for disorders with factitious symptoms that do not meet criteria for a specific Factitious Disorder.   For example, factitious disorder by proxy, i.e., the intentional production or feigning of physical signs or symptoms in another person who is under the individual's care for the purpose of indirectly assuming the sick role. (See page xx for suggested criteria).

Dissociative Disorders

300.12 Dissociative Amnesia

A. The predominant disturbance is one or more episodes of inability to recall important personal information, usually of a traumatic or stressful nature, that is too extensive to be explained by ordinary forgetfulness.

B. The disturbance does not occur exclusively during the course of Dissociative Identity Disorder and is not due to the direct effects of a substance (e.g., drugs of abuse, medication) or a general medical condition (e.g., Amnestic Disorder due to head trauma).

300.13 Dissociative Fugue

A. The predominant disturbance is sudden, unexpected travel away from home or one's customary place of work, with inability to recall one's past.

B. Confusion about personal identity or assumption of new identity (partial or complete).

C. The disturbance does not occur exclusively during the course of Dissociative Identity Disorder and is not due to the direct effects of a substance (e.g., drugs of abuse, medication) or a general medical condition (e.g., temporal lobe epilepsy).

300.14 Dissociative Identity Disorder (Multiple Personality Disorder)

A. The presence of two or more distinct identities or personality states (each with its own relatively enduring pattern of perceiving, relating to, and thinking about the environment and self).

B. At least two of these identities or personality states recurrently take control of the person's behavior.

C. Inability to recall important personal information that is too extensive to be explained by ordinary forgetfulness.

D. Not due to the direct effects of a substance (e.g., blackouts or chaotic behavior during Alcohol Intoxication) or a general medical condition (e.g., complex partial seizures).   Note: In children, the symptoms are not attributable to imaginary playmates or other fantasy play.

300.6 Depersonalization Disorder

A. Persistent or recurrent experiences of feeling detached from, and as if one is an outside observer of, one's mental processes or body (e.g., feeling like one is in a dream).

B. During the depersonalization experience, reality testing remains intact.

C. The depersonalization causes clinically significant distress or impairment in social, occupational, or other important areas of functioning.

D. The depersonalization experience is not better accounted for by another disorder, such as Schizophrenia, Dissociative Identity Disorder, or Panic Disorder, and is not due to the direct effects of a substance (e.g., drugs of abuse, medication) or a general medical condition (e.g., temporal lobe epilepsy).

300.15 Dissociative Disorder Not Otherwise Specified

This category is for disorders in which the predominant feature is a dissociative symptom (i.e., a disturbance or alteration in the normal integrative functions of identity, memory, or consciousness) but the criteria are not met for any specific Dissociative Disorder. Examples include:

1) Clinical presentations similar to Dissociative Identity Disorder that fail to meet full criteria for this disorder. Examples include presentations in which: (a) there are not two or more distinct personality states, or (b) amnesia for important personal information does not occur.

2) Derealization unaccompanied by depersonalization in adults.

3) States of dissociation that occur in individuals who have been subjected to periods of prolonged and intense coercive persuasion (e.g., brainwashing, thought reform, or indoctrination while the captive of terrorists or cultists).

4) Dissociative trance disorder: single or episodic alterations in the state of consciousness that are indigenous to particular locations and cultures. Dissociative trance involves narrowing of awareness of immediate surroundings or stereotyped behaviors or movements that are experienced as being beyond one's control. Possession trance involves replacement of the customary sense of personal identity by a new identity, attributed to the influence of a spirit, power, deity, or other person, and associated with stereotyped "involuntary" movements or amnesia. Examples include *amok* (Indonesia), *bebainan* (Indonesia), *latah* (Malaysia), *pibloktoq* (Artic), *phil pob* (Thailand), *vimbuza* (Nigeria), *ataque de nervios* (Latin America) and possession (India). The dissociative or trance disorder is not a normal part of a broadly accepted collective cultural or religious practice. (See page xx for suggested criteria).

5) Loss of consciousness, stupor, or coma not attributable to a general medical condition.

6) Ganser's syndrome: the giving of "appropriate answers" to questions, commonly associated with dissociative amnesia or fugue.

Sexual and Gender Identity Disorders

Sexual Dysfunctions

The following types apply to all the Sexual Dysfunctions:

Specify type:

Due to Psychological Factors or
Due to Combined Psychological Factors and a General Medical Condition

Lifelong (occurring during the person's entire sexual life) or **Acquired**

Generalized (occurring in all situations and with all partners) or **Situational**

Sexual Desire Disorders

302.71 Hypoactive Sexual Desire Disorder

A. Persistently or recurrently deficient (or absent) sexual fantasies and desire for sexual activity. The judgment of deficiency or absence is made by the clinician, taking into account factors that affect sexual functioning, such as age and the context of the person's life.

B. Does not occur exclusively during the course of another Axis I disorder (other than a Sexual Dysfunction), such as Major Depressive Disorder, and is not due to the direct effects of a substance (e.g., drugs of abuse, medication) or a general medical condition.

C. The disturbance causes marked distress or interpersonal difficulty.

302.79 Sexual Aversion Disorder

A. Persistent or recurrent extreme aversion to, and avoidance of all (or almost all), genital sexual contact with a sexual partner.

B. Does not occur exclusively during the course of another Axis I disorder (other than a Sexual Dysfunction) such as Obsessive-Compulsive Disorder or Major Depressive Disorder.

C. The disturbance causes marked distress or interpersonal difficulty.

Sexual Arousal Disorders

302.72 Female Sexual Arousal Disorder

A. Persistent or recurrent inability to attain or maintain an adequate lubrication-swelling response of sexual excitement until completion of the sexual activity.

B. Does not occur exclusively during the course of another Axis I disorder (other than a Sexual Dysfunction) such as Major Depressive Disorder, and is not due to the direct effects of a substance (e.g., drugs of abuse, medication) or a general medical condition.

C. The disturbance causes marked distress or interpersonal difficulty.

302.72 Male Erectile Disorder

A. Persistent or recurrent inability to attain or maintain an adequate erection until completion of the sexual activity.

B. Does not occur during the course of another Axis I disorder (other than a Sexual Dysfunction) such as Major Depressive Disorder, and is not due to the direct effects of a substance (e.g., drugs of abuse, medication) or a general medical condition.

C. The disturbance causes marked distress or interpersonal difficulty.

Orgasm Disorders

302.73 Female Orgasmic Disorder (Inhibited Female Orgasm)

A. Persistent or recurrent delay in, or absence of, orgasm following a normal sexual excitement phase. Women exhibit wide variability in the type or intensity of stimulation that triggers orgasm. The diagnosis of Female Orgasmic Disorder should be based on the clinician's judgment that the woman's orgasmic capacity is less than would be reasonable for her age, sexual experience, and the adequacy of sexual stimulation she receives.

B. Does not occur exclusively during the course of another Axis I disorder (other than a Sexual Dysfunction), such as Major Depressive Disorder, and is not due to the direct effects of a substance (e.g., drugs of abuse, medication) or a general medical condition.

C. The disturbance causes marked distress or interpersonal difficulty.

302.74 Male Orgasmic Disorder (Inhibited Male Orgasm)

A.   Persistent or recurrent delay in, or absence of, orgasm following a normal sexual excitement phase during sexual activity that the clinician, taking into account the person's age, judges to be adequate in focus, intensity, and duration.

B.   Does not occur exclusively during the course of another Axis I disorder (other than a Sexual Dysfunction), such as Major Depressive Disorder, and is not due to the direct effects of a substance (e.g., drugs of abuse, medication) or a general medical condition.

C.   The disturbance causes marked distress or interpersonal difficulty.

302.75 Premature Ejaculation

A.   Persistent or recurrent ejaculation with minimal sexual stimulation before, upon, or shortly after penetration and before the person wishes it. The clinician must take into account factors that affect duration of the excitement phase, such as age, novelty of the sexual partner or situation, and frequency of sexual activity.

B.   The disturbance causes marked distress or interpersonal difficulty.

Sexual Pain Disorders

302.76 Dyspareunia

A.   Recurrent or persistent genital pain in either a male or a female before, during, or after sexual intercourse.

B.   The disturbance is not caused exclusively by Vaginismus or lack of lubrication, is not better accounted for by another Axis I disorder (e.g., Somatization Disorder), and is not due to the direct effects of a substance (e.g., drugs of abuse, medication) or a general medical condition.

C.   The disturbance causes marked distress or interpersonal difficulty.

306.51 Vaginismus

A.   Recurrent or persistent involuntary spasm of the musculature of the outer third of the vagina that interferes with sexual intercourse.

B.   The disturbance is not better accounted for by another Axis I disorder (e.g., Somatization Disorder) and is not due to the direct effects of a substance (e.g., drugs of abuse, medication) or a general medical condition.

C.   The disturbance causes marked distress or interpersonal difficulty.

Sexual Dysfunction Due to a General Medical Condition

A.   Clinically significant sexual dysfunction that results in marked distress or
      interpersonal difficulty.

B.   There is evidence from the history, physical examination, or laboratory findings of a
      general medical condition judged to be etiologically related to the sexual
      dysfunction.

607.84 Male Erectile Disorder Due to a General Medical Condition: if male erectile
      dysfunction is the predominant feature.

---.--   Dyspareunia Due to a General Medical Condition: if pain associated with
      intercourse is the predominant feature.
Code: **625.0** in a female
          608.89 in a male

**608.89 Male Hypoactive Sexual Desire Disorder Due to a General Medical
      Condition**: if deficient or absent sexual desire is the predominant feature.

**625.8   Female Hypoactive Sexual Desire Disorder Due to a General Medical
      Condition**: if deficient or absent sexual desire is the predominant feature.

608.89 Other Male Sexual Dysfunction Due to a General Medical Condition: if some
      other feature is predominant (e.g., orgasmic disorder) or no feature
      predominates.

625.8   Other Female Sexual Dysfunction Due to a General Medical Condition: if
      some other feature is predominant (e.g., orgasmic disorder) or no feature
      predominates.

Substance-Induced Sexual Dysfunction

A.   Clinically significant sexual dysfunction that results in marked distress or
      interpersonal difficulty.

B.   There is evidence from the history, physical examination, or laboratory findings of
      substance intoxication or withdrawal, and the symptoms in A developed during, or
      within a month of, significant substance intoxication or withdrawal.

C.   The disturbance is not better accounted for by a Sexual Dysfunction that is not
      substance-induced.   Evidence that the symptoms are better accounted for by a
      Sexual Dysfunction that is not substance-induced might include: the symptoms
      precede the onset of the substance abuse or dependence; persist for a substantial
      period of time (e.g., about a month) after the cessation of acute withdrawal or
      severe intoxication; are substantially in excess of what would be expected given the
      character, duration, or amount of the substance used; or there is other evidence
      suggesting the existence of an independent non-substance-induced Sexual
      Dysfunction (e.g., a history of recurrent non-substance-related episodes).

Code: (Specific Substance) Sexual Dysfunction
(291.8 Alcohol, 292.89 Amphetamine [or Related Substance], 292.89 Cocaine, 292.89 Opioid, 292.89 Sedative, Hypnotic, Anxiolytic, 292.89 Other [or Unknown] Substance)

Coding note: also code substance-specific Intoxication or Withdrawal if criteria are met.

Specify if:
with impaired desire
with impaired arousal
with impaired orgasm
with sexual pain

Specify if
with onset during intoxication

302.70 Sexual Dysfunction Not Otherwise Specified

This category includes sexual dysfunctions that do not meet criteria for any specific Sexual Dysfunction. Examples include:

1)   no (or substantially diminished) subjective erotic feelings despite otherwise normal arousal and orgasm.

2)   situations in which the clinician has concluded that a sexual dysfunction is present but is unable to determine whether it is primary, due to a general medical condition, or substance-induced.

Paraphilias

302.4 Exhibitionism

A.   Over a period of at least six months, recurrent intense sexual urges and sexually arousing fantasies involving the exposure of one's genitals to an unsuspecting stranger.

B.   The person has acted on these urges, or is markedly distressed by them.

302.81 Fetishism

A.   Over a period of at least six months, recurrent intense sexual urges and sexually arousing fantasies involving the use of nonliving objects (e.g., female undergarments).

B.   The person has acted on these urges, or is markedly distressed by them.

C.   The fetish objects are not articles of female clothing used exclusively in cross-dressing (as in Transvestic Fetishism) or devices designed for the purpose of tactile genital stimulation (e.g., vibrator).

302.85 Frotteurism

A.   Over a period of at least six months, recurrent intense sexual urges and sexually arousing fantasies involving touching and rubbing against a nonconsenting person. It is the touching, not the coercive nature of the act, that is sexually exciting.

B.   The person has acted on these urges, or is markedly distressed by them.

302.2 Pedophilia

A.   Over a period of at least six months, recurrent intense sexual urges and sexually arousing fantasies involving sexual activity with a prepubescent child or children (generally age 13 or younger).

B.   The person has acted on these urges, or is markedly distressed by them.

C.   The person is at least 16 years old and at least 5 years older than the child or children in A

Note: Do not include a late adolescent involved in an ongoing sexual relationship with a 12- or 13-year-old.

Specify if
Sexually Attracted to Males
Sexually Attracted to Females
Sexually Attracted to Both

Specify if **limited to incest.**

Specify type: **exclusive type** (attracted only to children), or **nonexclusive type.**

302.83 Sexual Masochism

A.   Over a period of at least six months, recurrent intense sexual urges and sexually arousing fantasies involving the act (real, not simulated) of being humiliated, beaten, bound, or otherwise made to suffer.

B.   The person has acted on these urges, or is markedly distressed by them.

302.84 Sexual Sadism

A.   Over a period of at least six months, recurrent intense sexual urges and sexually arousing fantasies involving acts (real, not simulated) in which the psychological or physical suffering (including humiliation) of the victim is sexually exciting to the person.

B.   The person has acted on these urges, or is markedly distressed by them.

302.82 Voyeurism

A.   Over a period of at least six months, recurrent intense sexual urges and sexually arousing fantasies involving the act of observing an unsuspecting person who is naked, in the process of disrobing, or engaging in sexual activity.

B.   The person has acted on these urges, or is markedly distressed by them.

302.3 Transvestic Fetishism

A.   Over a period of at least six months, in a heterosexual male, recurrent intense sexual urges and sexually arousing fantasies involving cross-dressing.

B.   The person has acted upon these urges or is markedly distressed by them.

C.   Does not occur exclusively during the course of Gender Identity Disorder.

Specify if **With Gender Dysphoria**: if the person has persistent discomfort with gender role or identity.

302.9 Paraphilia Not Otherwise Specified

The category is for paraphilias that do not meet criteria for any of the specific Paraphilias. Examples include:

1) telephone scatalogia (lewdness) (See page xx for suggested criteria).
2) necrophilia (corpses)
3) partialism (exclusive focus on part of body)
4) zoophilia (animals)
5) coprophilia (feces)
6) klismaphilia (enemas)
7) urophilia (urine)

302.9 Sexual Disorder Not Otherwise Specified

This category is for a sexual disturbance that does not meet the criteria for any specific Sexual Disorder and is neither a dysfunction nor a paraphilia. Examples include:

1) marked feelings of inadequacy concerning sexual performance or other traits related to self-imposed standards of masculinity or femininity.

2) distress about a pattern of repeated sexual relationships involving a succession of lovers who are experienced by the individual only as things to be used.

3) persistent and marked distress about one's sexual orientation.

Gender Identity Disorders

---.-- Gender Identity Disorder

A. A strong and persistent cross-gender identification (not merely a desire for any perceived cultural advantages of being the other sex).

In children, manifested by at least four of the following:

(1) repeatedly stated desire to be, or insistence that he or she is, the other sex

(2) in boys, preference for cross-dressing or simulating female attire; in girls, insistence on wearing only stereotypical masculine clothing

(3) strong and persistent preferences for cross-sex roles in make-believe play or persistent fantasies of being the other sex

(4) intense desire to participate in the stereotypical games and pastimes of the other sex

(5) strong preference for playmates of the other sex

In adolescents and adults, manifested by symptoms such as a stated desire to be the other sex, frequent passing as the other sex, desire to live or be treated as the other sex, or the conviction that one has the typical feelings and reactions of the other sex.

B. Persistent discomfort with one's sex or sense of inappropriateness in the gender role of that sex.

In children, manifested by any of the following: in boys, assertion that his penis or testes are disgusting or will disappear or assertion that it would be better not to have a penis, or aversion toward rough-and-tumble play and rejection of male stereotypical toys, games, and activities; in girls, rejection of urinating in a sitting position or assertion that she does not want to grow breasts or menstruate, or marked aversion towards normative feminine clothing.

In adolescents and adults, manifested by symptoms such as preoccupation with getting rid of one's primary and secondary sex characteristics (e.g., request for hormones, surgery, or other procedures to physically alter sexual characteristics to simulate the other sex) or belief that one was born the wrong sex.

C. Not concurrent with a physical intersex condition.

D. The disturbance causes clinically significant distress or impairment in social, occupational, or other important areas of functioning.

Code based on current age:

302.6   **if in childhood**
302.85   **if adolescent or adult**

Specify if (for sexually mature individuals):
   Sexually Attracted to Males
   Sexually Attracted to Females
   Sexually Attracted to Both
   Sexually Attracted to Neither

302.6 Gender Identity Disorder Not Otherwise Specified

Disorders in gender identity that are not classifiable as a specific Gender Identity Disorder. Examples include:

1)   individuals with intersex conditions (e.g., androgen insensitivity syndrome or congenital adrenal hyperplasia) and gender dysphoria

2)   adults with transient, stress-related cross-dressing behavior.

3)   individuals who have a persistent preoccupation with castration or peotomy without a desire to acquire the sex characteristics of the other sex.

Eating Disorders

307.1 Anorexia Nervosa

A. Refusal to maintain body weight at or above a minimally normal weight for age and height (e.g., weight loss leading to maintenance of body weight less than 85% of that expected; or failure to make expected weight gain during period of growth, leading to body weight less than 85% of that expected).

B. Intense fear of gaining weight or becoming fat, even though underweight.

C. Disturbance in the way in which one's body weight or shape is experienced; undue influence of body weight or shape on self-evaluation, or denial of the seriousness of the current low body weight.

D. In post-menarchal females, amenorrhea, i.e., the absence of at least three consecutive menstrual cycles. (A woman is considered to have amenorrhea if her periods occur only following hormone, e.g., estrogen, administration.)

Specify type:
>   **Restricting type:** During the episode of Anorexia Nervosa, the person does not regularly engage in binge eating or purging behavior (i.e., self-induced vomiting or the misuse of laxatives or diuretics)
>
>   **Binge Eating/Purging type:** During the episode of Anorexia Nervosa, the person regularly engages in binge eating or purging behavior (i.e., self-induced vomiting or the misuse of laxatives or diuretics)

307.51 Bulimia Nervosa

A. Recurrent episodes of binge eating. An episode of binge eating is characterized by both of the following:

   (1) eating, in a discrete period of time (e.g., within any two hour period), an amount of food that is definitely larger than most people would eat during a similar period of time and under similar circumstances, and,

   (2) a sense of lack of control over eating during the episode (e.g., a feeling that one cannot stop eating or control what or how much one is eating)

B. Recurrent inappropriate compensatory behavior in order to prevent weight gain, such as: self-induced vomiting; misuse of laxatives, diuretics or other medications; fasting; or excessive exercise.

C. The binge eating and inappropriate compensatory behaviors both occur, on average, at least twice a week for three months.

D.   Self-evaluation is unduly influenced by body shape and weight.

E.   The disturbance does not occur exclusively during episodes of Anorexia Nervosa.

Specify type:
   Purging type: the person regularly engages in self-induced vomiting or the misuse of laxatives or diuretics.
   Nonpurging type: the person uses other inappropriate compensatory behaviors, such as fasting or excessive exercise, but does not regularly engage in self-induced vomiting or the misuse of laxatives or diuretics.

307.50 Eating Disorder Not Otherwise Specified

This category is for disorders of eating that do not meet the criteria for any specific Eating Disorder. Examples include:

1)   all of the criteria for Anorexia Nervosa are met except the individual has regular menses

2)   all of the criteria for Anorexia Nervosa are met except that, despite significant weight loss, the individual's current weight is in the normal range.

3)   all of the criteria for Bulimia Nervosa are met except binges occur at a frequency of less than twice a week or for a duration of less than three months

4)   an individual of normal body weight who regularly engages in inappropriate compensatory behavior after eating small amounts of food (e.g., self-induced vomiting after the consumption of two cookies)

5)   an individual who repeatedly chews and spits out, but does not swallow, large amounts of food.

6)   Binge eating disorder: recurrent episodes of binge eating in the absence of the inappropriate compensatory behaviors characteristic of Bulimia Nervosa (see page xx for suggested criteria).

Sleep Disorders

Primary Sleep Disorders

Dyssomnias

307.42 Primary Insomnia

A. The predominant complaint is difficulty initiating or maintaining sleep, or nonrestorative sleep, for at least one month

B. The sleep disturbance (or associated daytime fatigue) causes clinically significant distress or impairment in social, occupational, or other important areas of functioning.

C. The sleep disturbance does not occur exclusively during the course of a Circadian Rhythm Sleep Disorder, Narcolepsy, Breathing-Related Sleep Disorder, or a Parasomnia.

D. Does not occur exclusively during the course of another mental disorder (e.g., Major Depressive Disorder, Generalized Anxiety Disorder).

E. Not due to the direct effects of a substance (e.g., drugs of abuse, medication) or a general medical condition.

307.44 Primary Hypersomnia

A. The predominant complaint is excessive sleepiness for at least one month (or less if recurrent) as evidenced by either prolonged sleep episodes or daytime sleep episodes occurring almost daily.

B. The excessive sleepiness causes clinically significant distress or impairment in social, occupational, or other important areas of functioning.

C. Not better accounted for by insomnia and does not occur exclusively during the course of another Sleep Disorder (e.g., Narcolepsy, Circadian Rhythm Sleep Disorder, Breathing-Related Sleep Disorder, or a Parasomnia) and cannot be accounted for by an inadequate amount of sleep.

D. Does not occur exclusively during the course of another mental disorder.

E.   Not due to the direct effects of a substance (e.g., drugs of abuse, medication) or a general medical condition.

Specify if: **recurrent**: if there are periods of excessive sleepiness lasting at least three days occurring several times a year for at least two years.

347 Narcolepsy

A.   Irresistible attacks of refreshing sleep occurring daily over at least three months.

B.   Cataplexy (i.e., brief episodes of sudden bilateral loss of muscle tone, most often in association with intense emotion).

C.   Recurrent intrusions of elements of rapid eye movement (REM) sleep into the transition between sleep and wakefulness, as manifested by either hypnopompic/hypnogogic hallucinations or sleep paralysis at the beginning or end of sleep episodes.

D.   Not due to the direct effects of a substance (e.g., drugs of abuse, medication) or a general medical condition.

780.59 Breathing-Related Sleep Disorder

A.   Sleep disruption leading to excessive sleepiness or insomnia.

B.   The sleep disruption is judged to be due to a sleep-related breathing disorder (e.g., the sleep apnea or central alveolar hypoventilation syndrome).

C.   Not better accounted for by another mental disorder and not due to the direct effects of a substance (e.g., drugs of abuse, medication) or a general medical condition (other than a breathing-related disorder).

307.45 Circadian Rhythm Sleep Disorder (Sleep-Wake Schedule Disorder)

A.   A persistent or recurrent pattern of sleep disruption leading to excessive sleepiness or insomnia that is due to a mismatch between the sleep-wake schedule required by a person's environment and his or her circadian sleep-wake pattern.

B.   The sleep disturbance causes clinically significant distress or impairment in social, occupational, or other important areas of functioning.

C.   The disturbance does not occur exclusively during the course of another Sleep Disorder or other mental disorder.

D.   Not due to the direct effects of a substance (e.g., drugs of abuse, medication) or a general medical condition.

Specify type:
Delayed sleep phase type: A persistent pattern of late sleep onset and late awakening times, with an inability to fall asleep and awaken at a desired earlier time.
Jet lag type: Sleepiness and alertness that occur at an inappropriate time of day relative to local time, occurring after repeated travel across more than one time zone.
Shift work type: Insomnia during major sleep period or excessive sleepiness during major wake period associated with night-shift work or frequently changing shift work.
Unspecified.

307.47 Dyssomnia Not Otherwise Specified

This category is for insomnias, hypersomnias, or circadian rhythm disturbances that do not meet criteria for any specific Dyssomnia. Examples include:

1) nocturnal myoclonus: repeated limb jerks, particularly in the lower extremities, typically associated with brief periods of arousal.

2) situations in which the clinician has concluded that a Dyssomnia is present but is unable to determine whether it is primary, due to a general medical condition, or substance-induced.

Parasomnias

307.47 Nightmare Disorder (Dream Anxiety Disorder)

A.   Repeated awakenings from the major sleep period or naps with detailed recall of extended and extremely frightening dreams, usually involving threats to survival, security, or self-esteem. The awakenings generally occur during the second half of the sleep period.

B.   On awakening from the frightening dreams, the person rapidly becomes oriented and alert (in contrast to the confusion and disorientation seen in Sleep Terror Disorder and some forms of epilepsy).

C.   The dream experience, or the sleep disturbance resulting from the awakening, causes clinically significant distress or impairment in social, occupational, or other important areas of functioning.

D.   Not due to the direct effects of a substance (e.g., drugs of abuse, medication) or a general medical condition.

307.46 Sleep Terror Disorder

A.   Recurrent episodes of abrupt awakening from sleep, usually occurring during the first third of the major sleep episode and beginning with a panicky scream.

B.   Intense anxiety and signs of autonomic arousal during each episode, such as tachycardia, rapid breathing, and sweating.

C.   No detailed dream is recalled, and there is amnesia for the episode.

D.   Relative unresponsiveness to efforts of others to comfort the person during the episode.

E.   Not due to the direct effects of a substance (e.g., drugs of abuse, medication) or a general medical condition.

307.46 Sleepwalking Disorder

A.   Repeated episodes of arising from bed during sleep and walking about, usually occurring during the first third of the major sleep episode.

B.   While sleepwalking, the person has a blank, staring face, is relatively unresponsive to the efforts of others to communicate with him or her, and can be awakened only with great difficulty.

C. On awakening (either from the sleepwalking episode or the next morning), the person has amnesia for the episode.

D. Within several minutes after awakening from the sleepwalking episode, there is no impairment of mental activity or behavior (although there may initially be a short period of confusion or disorientation).

E. Not due to the direct effects of a substance (e.g., drugs of abuse, medication) or a general medical condition.

307.40 Parasomnia Not Otherwise Specified

This category is for disturbances during sleep that do not meet criteria for any specific Parasomnia. Examples include:

1) medical conditions exacerbated during sleep, e.g., nocturnal angina.

2) situations in which the clinician has concluded that a Parasomnia is present but is unable to determine whether it is primary, due to a general medical condition, or substance-induced.

Sleep Disorders Related to Another Mental Disorder

307.42 Insomnia Related to [Axis I or Axis II disorder]

A. The predominant complaint is difficulty initiating or maintaining sleep, or nonrestorative sleep, for at least one month.

B. The sleep disturbance is associated with daytime fatigue or impaired daytime functioning.

C. The sleep disturbance (or daytime sequelae) causes clinically significant distress or impairment in social, occupational, or other important areas of functioning.

D. The insomnia is judged to be related to another Axis I or Axis II disorder (e.g., Major Depressive Disorder, Generalized Anxiety Disorder, Adjustment Disorder with Anxiety) but is sufficiently severe to warrant independent clinical attention.

E. Not due to the direct effects of a substance (e.g., drugs of abuse, medication) or a general medical condition.

307.44 Hypersomnia Related to [Axis I or Axis II disorder]

A.   The predominant complaint is excessive sleepiness for at least one month as evidenced by either prolonged sleep episodes or daytime sleep episodes occurring almost daily.

B.   The excessive sleepiness causes clinically significant distress or impairment in social, occupational, or other important areas of functioning.

C.   The hypersomnia is judged to be related to another Axis I or Axis II disorder (e.g., Major Depressive Disorder, Dysthymic Disorder), but is sufficiently severe to warrant independent clinical attention.

D.   Not due to the direct effects of a substance (e.g., drugs of abuse, medication) or a general medical condition.

Other Sleep Disorders

780.5x Sleep Disorder Due to a General Medical Condition

A.   A prominent disturbance in sleep which is sufficiently severe to warrant independent clinical attention.

B.   There is evidence from the history, physical examination, or laboratory findings of a general medical condition judged to be etiologically related to the sleep disturbance.

C.   The sleep disturbance causes clinically significant distress or impairment in social, occupational, or other important areas of functioning.

D.   Does not meet criteria for a Breathing-related Sleep Disorder or Narcolepsy.

E.   Does not occur exclusively during the course of Delirium.

Specify type:
   .x2 **Insomnia Type:** if the predominant sleep disturbance is insomnia.
   .x4 **Hypersomnia Type:** if the predominant sleep disturbance is hypersomnia.
   .x9 **Parasomnia Type:** if the prominent sleep disturbance is a parasomnia.
   .x9 **Mixed Type:** if more than one sleep disturbance is present and none predominates.

Sleep Disorders

Substance-Induced Sleep Disorder

A.   A prominent disturbance in sleep which is sufficiently severe to warrant independent clinical attention.

B.   There is evidence from the history, physical examination, or laboratory findings of substance intoxication or withdrawal, and the symptoms in A developed during, or within a month of, significant substance intoxication or withdrawal.

C.   The disturbance is not better accounted for by a Sleep Disorder that is not substance-induced.   Evidence that the symptoms are better accounted for by a Sleep Disorder that is not substance-induced might include: the symptoms precede the onset of the substance abuse or dependence; persist for a substantial period of time (e.g., about a month) after the cessation of acute withdrawal or severe intoxication; are substantially in excess of what would be expected given the character, duration, or amount of the substance used; or there is other evidence suggesting the existence of an independent non-substance-induced disorder (e.g., history of recurrent non-substance-related episodes).

D.   The sleep disturbance causes clinically significant distress or impairment in social, occupational, or other important areas of functioning.

Code: (Specific Substance) Sleep Disorder
       (292.89 Alcohol, 292.89 Amphetamine [or Related Substance], 292.89 Caffeine, 292.89 Cocaine, 292.89 Opioid, 292.89 Sedative, Hypnotic, or Anxiolytic, 292.89 Other [or Unknown] Substance)

Coding note: also code substance-specific Intoxication or Withdrawal if criteria are met.

Specify if: (see table on page xx for applicability by substance)
       with onset during intoxication
       with onset during withdrawal

Specify type:
       Insomnia type: if the predominant sleep disturbance is insomnia.
       Hypersomnia type: if the predominant sleep disturbance is hypersomnia.
       Parasomnia type: if the prominent sleep disturbance is a parasomnia.
       Mixed type: if more than one sleep disturbance is present and none predominates.

Impulse Control Disorders Not Elsewhere Classified

312.34 Intermittent Explosive Disorder

A. Several discrete episodes of loss of control of aggressive impulses resulting in serious assaultive acts or destruction of property.

B. The degree of aggressiveness expressed during the episodes is grossly out of proportion to any precipitating psychosocial stressors.

C. The episodes of loss of control are not better accounted for by Antisocial Personality Disorder, Borderline Personality Disorder, a Psychotic disorder, a manic episode, Conduct Disorder, or Attention Deficit/Hyperactivity Disorder; and are not due to the direct effects of a substance (e.g., drugs of abuse, medication), or a general medical condition (e.g., Personality Change Due to Head Trauma).

312.32 Kleptomania

A. Recurrent failure to resist impulses to steal objects not needed for personal use or for their monetary value.

B. Increasing sense of tension immediately before committing the theft.

C. Pleasure, gratification, or relief at the time of committing the theft.

D. The stealing is not committed to express anger or vengeance, and is not in response to a delusion or hallucination.

E. The stealing is not better accounted for by a Conduct Disorder, manic episode, or Antisocial Personality Disorder.

312.33 Pyromania

A. Deliberate and purposeful fire setting on more than one occasion.

B. Tension or affective arousal before the act.

C. Fascination with, interest in, curiosity about, or attraction to fire and its situational contexts or associated characteristics (e.g., paraphernalia, uses, consequences, exposure to fires).

D. Pleasure, gratification, or relief when setting fires, or when witnessing or participating in their aftermath.

E.   The fire setting is not done for monetary gain, as an expression of sociopolitical ideology, to conceal criminal activity, to express anger or vengeance, to improve one's living circumstances, or in response to a delusion or hallucination.

F.   The fire setting is not better accounted for by Antisocial Personality Disorder, Conduct Disorder, or a manic episode.

312.31 Pathological Gambling

A.   Persistent and recurrent maladaptive gambling behavior as indicated by at least five of the following:

(1)   preoccupation with gambling (e.g., preoccupied with reliving past gambling experiences, handicapping or planning the next venture, or thinking of ways to get money with which to gamble)

(2)   the need to gamble with increasing amounts of money in order to achieve the desired excitement

(3)   repeated unsuccessful efforts to control, cut back, or stop gambling

(4)   restlessness or irritability when attempting to cut down or stop gambling

(5)   gambles as a way of escaping from problems or of relieving dysphoric mood (e.g., feelings of helplessness, guilt, anxiety, depression)

(6)   after losing money gambling, often returns another day in order to get even ("chasing" one's losses)

(7)   lies to family members, therapists, or others to conceal the extent of involvement with gambling

(8)   has committed illegal acts such as forgery, fraud, theft, or embezzlement, in order to finance gambling

(9)   has jeopardized or lost a significant relationship, job, or educational or career opportunity because of gambling

(10) reliance on others to provide money to relieve a desperate financial situation caused by gambling

B.   Is not better accounted for by a manic episode.

312.39 Trichotillomania

A. Recurrent pulling out of one's hair resulting in noticeable hair loss.

B. Increasing sense of tension immediately before pulling out the hair.

C. Pleasure, gratification, or relief when pulling out the hair.

D. Not better accounted for by another mental disorder and not to due to a general medical condition (e.g., a dermatologic disorder).

312.30 Impulse Control Disorder Not Otherwise Specified

This category is for disorders of impulse control that do not meet the criteria for any specific Impulse Control Disorder.

Adjustment Disorder

Adjustment Disorder

A. The development of emotional or behavioral symptoms in response to an identifiable stressor(s) occurring within three months of the onset of the stressor(s).

B. These symptoms or behaviors are clinically significant as evidenced by either of the following:

    (1) marked distress that is in excess of what would be expected from exposure to the stressor

    (2) significant impairment in social or occupational (academic) functioning

C. The stress-related disturbance does not meet the criteria for any specific Axis I disorder and is not merely an exacerbation of a preexisting Axis I or Axis II disorder.

D. Does not represent Bereavement.

E. The symptoms do not persist for more than six months after the termination of the stressor (or its consequences).

Specify if:
   Acute: if the symptoms have persisted for less than six months
   Chronic: if the symptoms have persisted for six months or longer

Code based on type:
   309.24 With Anxiety
   309.0   With Depressed Mood
   309.3   With Disturbance of Conduct
   309.4   With Mixed Disturbance of Emotions and Conduct
   309.28 With Mixed Anxiety and Depressed Mood
   309.9   Unspecified

Personality Disorders

Cluster A

301.0 Paranoid Personality Disorder

A.   A pervasive distrust and suspiciousness of others such that their motives are interpreted as malevolent, beginning by early adulthood and present in a variety of contexts, as indicated by at least four of the following:

   (1)   suspects, without sufficient basis, that others are exploiting or deceiving him or her

   (2)   preoccupied with unjustified doubts about the loyalty or trustworthiness of friends or associates

   (3)   is reluctant to confide in others because of unwarranted fear that the information will be used maliciously against him or her

   (4)   reads hidden demeaning or threatening meanings into benign remarks or events

   (5)   persistently bears grudges, i.e., is unforgiving of insults, injuries, or slights

   (6)   perceives attacks on his or her character or reputation that are not apparent to others and is quick to react angrily or to counterattack

   (7)   recurrent suspicions, without justification, regarding fidelity of spouse or sexual partner

B.   Does not occur exclusively during the course of Schizophrenia, a Mood Disorder With Psychotic Features, or another Psychotic Disorder, and is not due to the direct effects of a general medical condition.

   Note: if criteria are met prior to the onset of Schizophrenia, add "pre-morbid," e.g., "Paranoid Personality Disorder (pre-morbid)."

301.20 Schizoid Personality Disorder

A. A pervasive pattern of detachment from social relationships and a restricted range of expression of emotions in interpersonal settings, beginning by early adulthood and present in a variety of contexts, as indicated by at least four of the following:

    (1) neither desires nor enjoys close relationships, including being part of a family

    (2) almost always chooses solitary activities

    (3) little, if any, interest in having sexual experiences with another person

    (4) takes pleasure in few, if any, activities

    (5) lacks close friends or confidants other than first-degree relatives

    (6) appears indifferent to the praise or criticism of others

    (7) emotional coldness, detachment, or flattened affectivity

B. Does not occur exclusively during the course of Schizophrenia, a Mood Disorder With Psychotic Features, another Psychotic Disorder, or a Pervasive Developmental Disorder, and is not due to the direct effects of a general medical condition.

    Note: if criteria are met prior to the onset of Schizophrenia, add "pre-morbid," e.g., "Schizoid Personality Disorder (pre-morbid)."

301.22 Schizotypal Personality Disorder

A.   A pervasive pattern of social and interpersonal deficits marked by acute discomfort with, and reduced capacity for, close relationships as well as by cognitive or perceptual distortions and eccentricities of behavior, beginning by early adulthood and present in a variety of contexts, as indicated by at least five of the following:

   (1)   ideas of reference (excluding delusions of reference)

   (2)   odd beliefs or magical thinking that influence behavior and are inconsistent with subcultural norms (e.g., superstitiousness, belief in clairvoyance, telepathy, or "sixth sense;" in children and adolescents, bizarre fantasies or preoccupations)

   (3)   unusual perceptual experiences, including bodily illusions

   (4)   odd thinking and speech (e.g., vague, circumstantial, metaphorical, overelaborate, or stereotyped)

   (5)   suspiciousness or paranoid ideation

   (6)   inappropriate or constricted affect

   (7)   behavior or appearance that is odd, eccentric, or peculiar

   (8)   lacks close friends or confidants other than first-degree relatives

   (9)   excessive social anxiety that does not diminish with familiarity and tends to be associated with paranoid fears rather than negative judgments about self

B.   Does not occur exclusively during the course of Schizophrenia, a Mood Disorder With Psychotic Features, another Psychotic Disorder, or a Pervasive Developmental Disorder.

   Note: if criteria are met prior to the onset of Schizophrenia, add "pre-morbid," e.g., "Schizotypal Personality Disorder (pre-morbid)."

Cluster B

301.7 Antisocial Personality Disorder

A.   Current age at least 18 years.

B.   Evidence of Conduct Disorder with onset before age 15 (see page xx):

C.   A pervasive pattern of disregard for and violation of the rights of others occurring since age 15, as indicated by at least three of the following:

    (1)   failure to conform to social norms with respect to lawful behaviors as indicated by repeatedly performing acts that are grounds for arrest

    (2)   irritability and aggressiveness, as indicated by repeated physical fights or assaults

    (3)   consistent irresponsibility, as indicated by repeated failure to sustain consistent work behavior or honor financial obligations

    (4)   impulsivity or failure to plan ahead

    (5)   deceitfulness, as indicated by repeated lying, use of aliases, or conning others for personal profit or pleasure.

    (6)   reckless disregard for safety of self or others.

    (7)   lack of remorse, as indicated by being indifferent to or rationalizing having hurt, mistreated, or stolen from another

D.   Occurrence of antisocial behavior is not exclusively during the course of Schizophrenia or a manic episode.

301.83 Borderline Personality Disorder

A pervasive pattern of instability of interpersonal relationships, self-image, affects, and control over impulses beginning by early adulthood and present in a variety of contexts, as indicated by at least five of the following:

(1) frantic efforts to avoid real or imagined abandonment. Note: do not include suicidal or self-mutilating behavior covered in criterion (5)

(2) a pattern of unstable and intense interpersonal relationships characterized by alternating between extremes of idealization and devaluation

(3) identity disturbance: persistent and markedly disturbed, distorted, or unstable self-image or sense of self

(4) impulsivity in at least two areas that are potentially self-damaging (e.g., spending, sex, substance abuse, reckless driving, binge eating). Note: do not include suicidal or self-mutilating behavior covered in criterion (5)

(5) recurrent suicidal behavior, gestures, or threats, or self-mutilating behavior

(6) affective instability due to a marked reactivity of mood (e.g., intense episodic dysphoria, irritability, or anxiety usually lasting a few hours and only rarely more than a few days)

(7) chronic feelings of emptiness

(8) inappropriate, intense anger or lack of control of anger (e.g., frequent displays of temper, constant anger, recurrent physical fights)

(9) transient, stress-related paranoid ideation or severe dissociative symptoms

301.50 Histrionic Personality Disorder

A pervasive pattern of excessive emotionality and attention seeking, beginning by early adulthood and present in a variety of contexts, as indicated by at least five of the following:

(1) is uncomfortable in situations in which he or she is not the center of attention

(2) interaction with others is often characterized by inappropriate sexually seductive or provocative behavior

(3) displays rapidly shifting and shallow expression of emotions

(4) consistently uses physical appearance to draw attention to oneself

(5) style of speech that is excessively impressionistic and lacking in detail

(6) self-dramatization, theatricality, and exaggerated expression of emotion

(7) suggestibility, i.e., easily influenced by others or circumstances

(8) considers relationships to be more intimate than they actually are

301.81 Narcissistic Personality Disorder

A pervasive pattern of grandiosity (in fantasy or behavior), need for admiration, and lack of empathy, beginning by early adulthood and present in a variety of contexts, as indicated by at least five of the following:

(1) a grandiose sense of self-importance (e.g., exaggerates achievements and talents, expects to be recognized as superior without commensurate achievements)

(2) preoccupation with fantasies of unlimited success, power, brilliance, beauty, or ideal love

(3) believes that he or she is "special" and unique and can only be understood by, or should associate with, other special or high-status people (or institutions)

(4) requires excessive admiration

(5) a sense of entitlement i.e., unreasonable expectations of especially favorable treatment or automatic compliance with his or her expectations

(6) is interpersonally exploitative i.e., takes advantage of others to achieve his or her own ends

(7) lack of empathy: unwilling to recognize or identify with the feelings and needs of others

(8) is often envious of others or believes that others are envious of him or her

(9) arrogant, haughty behaviors or attitudes

Cluster C

301.82 Avoidant Personality Disorder

A pervasive pattern of social inhibition, feelings of inadequacy, and hypersensitivity to negative evaluation, beginning by early adulthood and present in a variety of contexts, as indicated by at least four of the following:

(1)   avoids occupational activities that involve significant interpersonal contact, because of fears of criticism, disapproval, or rejection

(2)   is unwilling to get involved with people unless certain of being liked

(3)   restraint within intimate relationships due to the fear of being shamed or ridiculed.

(4)   preoccupation with being criticized or rejected in social situations

(5)   inhibited in new interpersonal situations because of feelings of inadequacy

(6)   belief that one is socially inept, personally unappealing, or inferior to others

(7)   is unusually reluctant to take personal risks or to engage in any new activities because they may prove embarrassing

301.6 Dependent Personality Disorder

A pervasive and excessive need to be taken care of, leading to submissive and clinging behavior and fears of separation, beginning by early adulthood and present in a variety of contexts, as indicated by at least five of the following:

(1)   is unable to make everyday decisions without an excessive amount of advice and reassurance from others

(2)   needs others to assume responsibility for most major areas of his or her life

(3)   has difficulty expressing disagreement with others because of fear of loss of support or approval (Note: do not include realistic fears of retribution)

(4)   has difficulty initiating projects or doing things on his or her own (due to a lack of self-confidence in judgment or abilities rather than to a lack of motivation or energy)

(5)   goes to excessive lengths to obtain nurturance and support from others, to the point of volunteering to do things that are unpleasant

(6)   feels uncomfortable or helpless when alone, because of exaggerated fears of being unable to care for himself or herself

(7)   urgently seeks another relationship as a source of care and support when a close relationship ends

(8)   unrealistic preoccupation with fears of being left to take care of himself or herself

301.4 Obsessive-Compulsive Personality Disorder

A pervasive pattern of preoccupation with orderliness, perfectionism, and mental and interpersonal control, at the expense of flexibility, openness, and efficiency, beginning by early adulthood and present in a variety of contexts, as indicated by at least four of the following:

(1) preoccupation with details, rules, lists, order, organization, or schedules to the extent that the major point of the activity is lost

(2) perfectionism that interferes with task completion (e.g., inability to complete a project because one's own overly strict standards are not met)

(3) excessive devotion to work and productivity to the exclusion of leisure activities and friendships (not accounted for by obvious economic necessity)

(4) overconscientiousness, scrupulousness, and inflexibility about matters of morality, ethics, or values (not accounted for by cultural or religious identification)

(5) inability to discard worn-out or worthless objects even when they have no sentimental value

(6) reluctant to delegate tasks or to work with others unless they submit to exactly his or her way of doing things

(7) adopts a miserly spending style toward both self and others; money is viewed as something to be hoarded for future catastrophes

(8) rigidity and stubbornness

301.9 Personality Disorder Not Otherwise Specified

This category is for disorders of personality functioning that do not meet criteria for any specific Personality Disorder. An example is the presence of features of more than one specific Personality Disorder that do not meet the full criteria for any one Personality Disorder, but together cause clinically significant distress or impairment in one or more important areas of functioning (e.g., social or occupational). This category can also be used when the clinician judges that a specific Personality Disorder not included in this classification is appropriate. Examples include Passisve Aggressive Personality Disorder and (?) Depressive Personality Disorder (see page xx for suggested criteria).

Other Conditions That May Be a Focus of Clinical Attention

This section covers other conditions or problems that may be a focus of clinical attention that are available for coding on Axis I. These problems may be related to the mental disorders described previously in this manual in one of the following ways: 1) the problem is the focus of diagnosis or treatment and the individual has no mental disorder (e.g., Partner Relational Problem in which neither partner meets criteria for a mental disorder); 2) the individual has a mental disorder but it is unrelated to the problem (e.g., Partner Relational Problem in which one of the partners has an incidental Specific Phobia; 3) the individual has a mental disorder that is related to the problem, but the problem is sufficiently severe to warrant independent clinical attention (e.g., Partner Relational Problem associated with Major Depressive Disorder in one of the partners, that is sufficiently problematic to be a focus of treatment).

PSYCHOLOGICAL FACTORS AFFECTING MEDICAL CONDITION

316 Psychological Factors Affecting Medical Condition

A.   The presence of a general medical condition (coded on Axis III)

B.   Psychological factors adversely affect the general medical condition in one of the following ways:

(1)   the factors have influenced the course of the general medical condition as shown by a close temporal association between the psychological factors and the development or exacerbation of, or delayed recovery from, the general medical condition.

(2)   the factors interfere with the treatment of the general medical condition.

(3)   the factors constitute additional health risks for the individual.

(4)   the factors elicit stress-related physiologic responses that precipitate or exacerbate symptoms of a general medical condition (e.g., chest pain or arrhythmia in a patient with coronary artery disease)

Choose name based on the nature of the psychological factors: (if more than one factor is present, indicate the most prominent)

Mental Disorder Affecting Medical Condition (e.g., an Axis I disorder such as Major Depressive Disorder delaying recovery from a myocardial infarction)
Psychological Symptoms Affecting Medical Condition (e.g., depressive symptoms delaying recovery from surgery; anxiety exacerbating asthma)
Personality Traits or Coping Style Affecting Medical Condition (e.g., pathological denial of the need for surgery in a patient with cancer; hostile, pressured behavior contributing to cardiovascular disease)
Maladaptive Health Behaviors Affecting Medical Condition (e.g., non-compliance with medication or diet; overeating)
Unspecified Psychological Factors Affecting Medical Condition

MEDICATION-INDUCED MOVEMENT DISORDERS

The following medication-induced movement disorders are included because of their frequent importance in: 1) the management of individuals treated with medication for mental disorders; and 2) the differential diagnosis with Axis I disorders (e.g., Anxiety Disorder vs. Neuroleptic-induced Akathisia, catatonia vs. Neuroleptic Malignant Syndrome). Medication-induced movement disorders should be coded on Axis I. Although these disorders are labelled "medication-induced," it is often difficult to establish the causal relationship between medication exposure and the development of the movement disorder especially since some of these movement disorders occur in the absence of medication exposure.

332.1 Neuroleptic-induced Parkinsonism

Parkinsonian tremor, muscular rigidity or akinesia developing within a few weeks of starting or raising the dose of a neuroleptic medication, or reducing medication used to treat extrapyramidal symptoms. (See page xx for suggested criteria).

333.92 Neuroleptic Malignant Syndrome

Severe muscle rigidity, elevated temperature, and other related findings (e.g., diaphoresis, dysphagia, incontinence, changes in level of consciousness ranging from confusion to coma, mutism, elevated or labile blood pressure, elevated CPK) developing in association with the use of neuroleptic medication. (See page xx for suggested criteria).

333.7 Neuroleptic-induced Acute Dystonia

Abnormal positioning or spasm of the muscles of the head, neck, limbs, or trunk developing within a few days of starting or raising the dose of a neuroleptic medication, or reducing medication used to treat extrapyramidal symptoms. (See page xx for suggested criteria).

333.99 Neuroleptic-induced Acute Akathisia

Subjective complaints of restlessness accompanied by observed movements (e.g., fidgety movements of the legs, rocking from foot to foot, pacing, or inability to sit or stand still) developing within a few weeks of starting or raising the dose of a neuroleptic medication, or reducing medication used to treat extrapyramidal symptoms. (See page xx for suggested criteria).

333.82 Neuroleptic-induced Tardive Dyskinesia

Involuntary choreiform, athetoid, or rhythmic movements (lasting at least a few weeks) of the tongue, jaw, or extremities developing in association with the use of neuroleptic medication for at least a few months (may be for a shorter period of time in the elderly). (See page xx for suggested criteria).

333.1 Medication-induced Postural Tremor

Fine tremor occurring during attempts to maintain a posture and developing in association with the use of medication, e.g., lithium, antidepressants, valproate. (See page xx for suggested criteria).

333.90 Medication-induced Movement Disorder Not Otherwise Specified.

This category is for medication-induced movement disorders not classified by any of the specific disorders listed above. Examples include parkinsonism, acute akathisia, acute dystonia, dyskinetic movement, or a neuroleptic malignant syndrome-like presentation associated with a medication other than a neuroleptic; tardive dystonia.

995.2 Adverse Effects of Medication Not Otherwise Specified

This category is available for optional use by clinicians to code side effects of medication (other than movement symptoms) when these adverse effects become a main focus of clinical attention. Examples include: severe hypotension, cardiac arrhythmias, and priapism.

RELATIONAL PROBLEMS

V61.9 Relational Problem Related to A Mental Disorder or General Medical Condition

This category should be used when the focus of clinical attention is a pattern of impaired interaction associated with a mental disorder or a general medical condition in a family member.

V61.20 Parent-Child Relational Problem

This category should be used when the focus of clinical attention is a pattern of interaction between parent and child (e.g., impaired communication, overprotection, inadequate discipline) associated with clinically significant impairment in individual or family functioning or clinically significant symptoms.

V61.12 Partner Relational Problem

This category should be used when the focus of clinical attention is a pattern of interaction between spouses or partners characterized by negative communication (e.g., criticisms), distorted communication (e.g., unrealistic expectations) or non-communication (e.g., withdrawal) associated with clinically significant impairment in individual or family functioning or symptoms in one or both partners.

V61.8 Sibling Relational Problem

This category should be used when the focus of clinical attention is a pattern of interaction between siblings associated with clinically significant impairment in individual or family functioning or symptoms in one or more of the siblings.

V62.81 Relational Problem Not Otherwise Specified

This category should be used when the focus of clinical attention is on relational problems not classifiable by any of the specific problems listed above. Example: difficulties with coworkers

PROBLEMS RELATED TO ABUSE OR NEGLECT

V61.21 Physical Abuse of Child

This category should be used when the focus of clinical attention is physical abuse of a child.

V61.22 Sexual Abuse of Child

This category should be used when the focus of clinical attention is sexual abuse of a child.

V61.21 Neglect of Child

This category should be used when the focus of clinical attention is child neglect.

V61.10 Physical Abuse of Adult

This category should be used when the focus of clinical attention is physical abuse of an adult (e.g., spouse beating, abuse of elderly parent).

V61.11 Sexual Abuse of Adult

This category should be used when the focus of clinical attention is sexual abuse of an adult (e.g., sexual coercion, rape).

ADDITIONAL CONDITIONS THAT MAY BE A FOCUS OF CLINICAL ATTENTION

V62.82 Bereavement

This category can be used when the focus of clinical attention is a reaction to the death of a loved one. As part of their reaction to the loss, some grieving individuals present with symptoms characteristic of a major depressive episode (e.g., feelings of sadness and associated symptoms such as insomnia, poor appetite, and weight loss). Certain symptoms are not characteristic of a "normal" grief reaction and may be helpful in differentiating bereavement from a major depressive episode. These include: 1) guilt about things other than actions taken or not taken by the survivor at the time of the death; 2) thoughts of death other than the survivor feeling that he or she would be better off dead or should have died with the deceased person; 3) morbid preoccupation with worthlessness; 4) marked psychomotor retardation; 5) prolonged and marked functional impairment; and 6) hallucinatory experiences other than thinking that he or she hears the voice of, or transiently sees the image of the deceased. The bereaved individual who does not have Major Depressive Disorder typically regards his or her depressed mood as "normal," although he or she may seek professional help for relief of such associated symptoms as insomnia or anorexia.

The duration of "normal" bereavement varies considerably among different cultural groups. The diagnosis of Major Depressive Disorder is generally not given unless the symptoms are still present two months after the loss.

V40.0 Borderline Intellectual Functioning

This category can be used when the focus of attention or treatment is associated with borderline intellectual functioning, i.e., an IQ in the 71-84 range. Differential diagnosis between Borderline Intellectual Functioning and Mental Retardation (an IQ of 70 or below) is especially difficult and important when the coexistence of certain mental disorders is involved. For example, when the diagnosis is Schizophrenia, Undifferentiated or Residual Type, and impairment in adaptive functioning is prominent, the existence of Borderline Intellectual Functioning is easily overlooked, and hence the level and quality of potential adaptive functioning may be incorrectly assessed.

V62.3 Academic Problem

This category can be used when the focus of attention or treatment is an academic problem that is not due to a mental disorder, or if due to a mental disorder, is sufficiently severe to warrant independent clinical attention. An example is a pattern of failing grades or of significant underachievement in a person with adequate intellectual capacity in the absence of a Learning or Communication Disorder or any other mental disorder that would account for the problem.

V62.2 Occupational Problem

This category can be used when the focus of attention or treatment is an occupational problem that is not due to a mental disorder, or if it is due to a mental disorder, is sufficiently severe to warrant independent clinical attention. Examples include job dissatisfaction and uncertainty about career choices.

V71.02 Childhood or Adolescent Antisocial Behavior

This category can be used when the focus of attention or treatment is antisocial behavior in a child or adolescent that is not due to a mental disorder (e.g., Conduct Disorder or an Impulse Control Disorder). Examples include isolated antisocial acts of children or adolescents (not a pattern of antisocial behavior).

V71.01 Adult Antisocial Behavior

This category can be used when the focus of attention or treatment is adult antisocial behavior that is not due to a mental disorder (e.g., Conduct Disorder, Antisocial Personality Disorder, or an Impulse Control Disorder). Examples include the behavior of some professional thieves, racketeers, or dealers in illegal substances.

V65.2 Malingering

The essential feature of Malingering is the intentional production of false or grossly exaggerated physical or psychological symptoms, motivated by external incentives such as avoiding military duty, avoiding work, obtaining financial compensation, evading criminal prosecution, or obtaining drugs. Under some circumstances Malingering may represent adaptive behavior, for example, feigning illness while a captive of the enemy during wartime.

Malingering should be strongly suspected if any combination of the following is noted:

(1) medicolegal context of presentation, e.g., the person is referred by his or her attorney to the physician for examination;
(2) marked discrepancy between the person's claimed stress or disability and the objective findings;
(3) lack of cooperation during the diagnostic evaluation and in complying with the prescribed treatment regimen;
(4) the presence of Antisocial Personality Disorder.

Malingering differs from Factitious Disorder in that the motivation for the symptom production in Malingering is an external incentive, whereas in Factitious Disorder there is an absence of external incentives. Evidence of an intrapsychic need to maintain the sick role suggests Factitious Disorder.

Malingering is differentiated from Conversion and other Somatoform Disorders by the intentional production of symptoms and by the obvious, external incentives. The person who is malingering is much less likely to present his or her symptoms in the context of emotional conflict, and the presenting symptoms are less likely to be related to an underlying emotional conflict. In Malingering (in contrast to Conversion Disorder), symptom relief is not often obtained by suggestion, hypnosis, or an amobarbital interview.

V62.89 Phase of Life Problem

This category can be used when the focus of attention or treatment is a problem associated with a particular developmental phase or some other life circumstance that is not due to a mental disorder, or if it is due to a mental disorder, is sufficiently severe to warrant independent clinical attention. Examples include problems associated with entering school, leaving parental control, starting a new career, and changes involved in marriage, divorce, and retirement.

V15.81 Noncompliance with Treatment for a Mental Disorder

This category can be used when the focus of attention or treatment is noncompliance with an important aspect of the treatment for a mental disorder. Examples include: irrationally motivated noncompliance due to denial of illness and decisions based on personal value judgments about the advantages and disadvantages of the proposed treatment.

313.82 Identity Problem

This category can be used when there is severe distress regarding uncertainty about issues relating to identity such as long-term goals, career choice, friendship patterns, sexual orientation and behavior, moral values, and group loyalties.

V62.61 Religious or Spiritual Problem

This category can be used when the focus of clinical attention is a religious or spiritual problem. Examples include distressing experiences that involve loss or questioning of faith, problems associated with conversion to a new faith, or questioning of other spiritual values which may not necessarily be related to an organized church or religious institution.

V62.4 Acculturation Problem

This category can be used when the focus of clinical attention is a problem involving adjustment to a different culture (e.g., following migration, social transplantation).

780.9 Age-Associated Memory Decline

This category can be used when the focus of clinical attention is a decline in memory consequent to the aging process that is within normal limits given the person's age. This code should only be considered after it has been determined that the memory decline is not attributable to a medical or neurological condition, e.g. Dementia.

Additional Codes

300.9 Unspecified Mental Disorder

There are several circumstances where it may be appropriate to assign this code: 1) for a specific mental disorder not included in the DSM-IV classification; 2) when none of the available Not Otherwise Specified categories is appropriate; 3) when it is judged that a mental disorder is present but there is not enough information available to diagnose one of the categories provided in classification. In some cases, the diagnosis can be changed to a specific disorder after more information is obtained.

V71.09 No Diagnosis or Condition on Axis I

When no Axis I diagnosis or condition is present, this should be indicated. There may or may not be an Axis II diagnosis.

799.9 Diagnosis or Condition Deferred on Axis I

When there is insufficient information to make any diagnostic judgment about an Axis I diagnosis or condition, this should be noted as Diagnosis or Condition Deferred on Axis I.

V71.09 No Diagnosis on Axis II

When no Axis II diagnosis (i.e., no Personality Disorder) is present, this should be indicated. There may or may not be an Axis I diagnosis or condition.

799.9 Diagnosis Deferred on Axis II

When there is insufficient information to make any diagnostic judgment about an Axis II diagnosis, this should be noted as Diagnosis Deferred on Axis II.

DSM-IV Appendices

Appendix A: Diagnostic Decision Trees

Appendix B: Criteria Sets and Axes Provided for Further Study

This Appendix contains a number of proposals for new categories and axes that were suggested for possible inclusion in DSM-IV. The DSM-IV Task Force and Work Groups subjected each of these proposals to a careful empirical review and invited wide commentary from the field. The Task Force determined that there was insufficient information to warrant inclusion of these proposals as official categories in DSM-IV. Text and criteria will be provided to facilitate systematic clinical research.

Asperger's disorder (if not included in the classification)
Postconcussional disorder
Mild cognitive disorder
Caffeine withdrawal
Postpsychotic depression of schizophrenia
Simple schizophrenia
Minor depressive disorder
Recurrent brief depressive disorder
Premenstrual dysphoric disorder
Mixed anxiety-depressive disorder
Factitious disorder by proxy
Dissociative trance disorder
Telephone scatalogia
Binge eating disorder
Depressive personality disorder (not yet decided whether to include in Appendix)
Passive aggressive personality disorder (Negativistic personality disorder)
Medication-induced Movement Disorders
      Neuroleptic-induced Parkinsonism
      Neuroleptic Malignant Syndrome
      Neuroleptic-induced Acute Dystonia
      Neuroleptic-induced Acute Akathisia
      Neuroleptic-induced Tardive Dyskinesia
      Medication-induced Postural Tremor
Axis for defense mechanisms
GARF (Global assessment of relational functioning scale)
SOFAS (Social and occupational functioning assessment scale)

Appendix C: Glossary of Technical Terms

Appendix D: Annotated Comparative Listing Between DSM-IV/DSM-III-R

Appendix E: Numeric Listing of DSM-IV Diagnoses and Codes (including E codes for noting specific substances)

Appendix F: Alphabetic Listing of DSM-IV Diagnoses and Codes

Appendix G: Selected ICD-9-CM Codes for General Medical Conditions

Appenidx H: Corresponding ICD-10 Codes for DSM-IV Disorders

Appendix I: Culturally-Related Syndromes

Appendix J: List of DSM-IV Participants.

Afterword

These <u>DSM-IV Draft Criteria</u> appear as we complete our work on DSM-IV. We have invited wide participation in the preparation of DSM-IV in order to produce a document which is not only empirically sound but is also sensitive to the many different needs of those who use the DSM. Interested readers can help us by calling to our attention any mistakes, inconsistencies, oversights, unforeseen problems, potentials for misuse or boundary confusions. Please send any comments to Dr. Allen Frances at the American Psychiatric Association, 1400 K Street, N.W., Washington, D.C. 20005.